Endoscopy for the veterinary technician

Endoscopy for the veterinary technician

EDITED BY

Susan Cox, RVT, VTS (SAIM)

Veterinary Technician
Small Animal Medicine Service
William R. Pritchard Veterinary Medical Teaching Hospital
University of California–Davis
Davis, California, USA

WILEY Blackwell

This edition first published 2016 © 2016 by John Wiley & Sons, Inc.

Editorial offices: 1606 Golden Aspen Drive, Suites 103 and 104, Ames, Iowa 50010, USA
The Atrium, Southern Gate, Chichester, West Sussex, PO19 8SQ, UK
9600 Garsington Road, Oxford, OX4 2DQ, UK

For details of our global editorial offices, for customer services and for information about how to apply for permission to reuse the copyright material in this book please see our website at www.wiley.com/wiley-blackwell.

Library of Congress Cataloging-in-Publication Data

Cox, Susan (Veterinary technician), author.
    Endoscopy for the veterinary technician / Susan Cox.
        p. ; cm.
    Includes bibliographical references and index.
    ISBN 978-1-118-43445-1 (pbk.)
    I. Title.
    [DNLM: 1. Endoscopy–methods. 2. Endoscopy–veterinary. 3. Animal Technicians.
4. Endoscopes–veterinary. SF 772.55]
    SF772.55.C68 2015
    636.089'705–dc23
                                                    2015018496

A catalogue record for this book is available from the British Library.

Wiley also publishes its books in a variety of electronic formats. Some content that appears in print may not be available in electronic books.

Set in 9.5/13 pt, MeridienLTStd by SPi Global, Chennai, India

Printed and bound in Malaysia by Vivar Printing Sdn Bhd

1   2016

Contents

List of contributors

Susan Cox, RVT, VTS (SAIM)
Veterinary Technician, Small Animal Medicine Service, William R. Pritchard Veterinary Medical Teaching Hospital, University of California–Davis, Davis, California, USA

Katie Douthitt, RVT
Small Animal Internal Medicine, William R. Pritchard Veterinary Medical Teaching Hospital, University of California–Davis, Davis, California, USA

Jody Nugent-Deal, RVT, VTS (Anes) (CP–Exotics)
Supervisor – Small Animal Anesthesia Department, William R. Pritchard Veterinary Medical Teaching Hospital, University of California–Davis, Davis, California, USA

Valerie Walker, RVT
Small Animal Internal Medicine, William R. Pritchard Veterinary Medical Teaching Hospital, University of California–Davis, Davis, California, USA

Introduction

My first exposure to veterinary endoscopy began with biopsy sampling only. I was not allowed to clean or even handle the endoscope – the busy internist insisted on performing these tasks between other procedures and appointments. This arrangement was not a very effective use of the technical staff, or benefited his busy schedule. Additionally, many technicians I have encountered are responsible for their clinic's endoscopes, with no idea of how to care for them properly. So my goal in writing this book was to give the endoscopy assistant the skills and knowledge to perform all facets of endoscope care and handling – before, during and after the procedure.

Many clinics are incorporating endoscopy into their hospitals as a minimally invasive medical instrument that can provide diagnostic and therapeutic options for treatment. Whether used in fluoroscopy, in the surgical suite, or in the treatment area, technical staff that are proficient in all aspects of endoscopy are invaluable.

Veterinary endoscopy textbooks are geared for the veterinary endoscopist and have little information regarding proper cleaning, disinfection, and instrumentation. These topics are fully covered here in Chapters 1 and 2, with tables that can be easily referenced during the cleaning process. Chapter 3 discusses the anesthetic challenges that patients undergoing endoscopic procedures can demonstrate, and how to address them. The next seven chapters provide a framework for preparation of the patient and procedure, specific instrumentation that will be needed, a navigational guide through a typical procedure, biopsy sampling and post-procedure patient care. The last chapter reviews the endoscopy suite, including equipment placement and organization.

I encourage all endoscopy assistants to attend wet labs and workshops with their endoscopists. More experience with basic techniques and learning new skills will enhance the reader's understanding of this text, and make the endoscopy assistant a more valued member of the endoscopy team!

Susan Cox

1 Endoscopy equipment

Valerie Walker

William R. Pritchard Veterinary Medical Teaching Hospital, University of California–Davis, Davis, California, USA

The endoscope is a medical instrument used for the visual examination of a body cavity or a hollow organ such as the lung, abdomen, ileum, colon, bladder, duodenum, nasal passages, or stomach. It is a rigid or flexible hollow tube fitted with a lens system and/or fiber-optic bundles to aid in the diagnosis and potential treatment of the patient. The function of the endoscope is to allow visualization of the mucosal surface to assess the degree of disease and allow tissue sampling for histopathology, culture, and cytology.

Endoscopy procedures have been a part of veterinary medicine since the 1970s. Today, these procedures are routinely performed in veterinary practices throughout the world. Types include bronchoscopy, esophagoscopy, gastroduodenoscopy, colonoscopy, nasopharyngoscopy, rhinoscopy, laparoscopy, and arthroscopy.

ENDOSCOPES

Endoscopes are manufactured in a variety of sizes with different function capabilities, depending on the needs of the endoscopist. Endoscopes are divided into two groups: rigid and flexible. Both types of endoscopes start with the construction of a hollow tube. To drive light through the endoscope, thin fiber-optic filaments assembled into bundles are used to transmit light (non-coherent), and the image (coherent) to the distal tip. The different uses of fiber-optics in endoscopes include the way in which images are transmitted back to the endoscopist and the functional characteristics of the endoscope. While all-fiber-optic endoscopes use coherent fiber-optic bundles to transmit the image, video endoscopes use a video chip and rigid telescopes utilize a lens/rod system.

Endoscopy for the Veterinary Technician, First Edition. Edited by Susan Cox.
© 2016 John Wiley & Sons, Inc. Published 2016 by John Wiley & Sons, Inc.

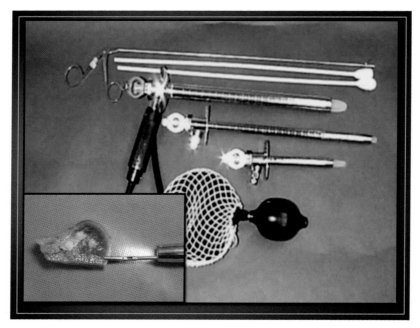

Figure 1.1 Sigmoidoscope with (from top) rigid biopsy forceps, large cotton tip applicators, sigmoidoscope with light handle and obturator. Inset: example of foreign body retrieved.

Rigid Endoscopes

Rigid endoscopes include sigmoidoscopes, pictured in Figure 1.1, and telescopes. The sigmoidoscope is used for visualization of the descending colon and rectum, and can be used in the esophagus to aid in the removal of foreign bodies. The sigmoidoscope is a hollow tube that can range from 10 to 19 mm in outer diameter (o.d.) with a length of 5–25 cm. When the viewing window is closed and the bulb insufflator engaged, a luminal view is obtained. Visualization is magnified through the lens of the viewing window and light is transmitted through fiber-optic bundles that encircle the inner recesses of the tube. Owing to the large inner diameter, multiple types of biopsy and retrieval forceps may be inserted when the viewing window is opened.

Telescopes are a higher quality medical-grade rigid endoscope. The hollow tube houses a series of glass rod lenses that magnify the image back to the eyepiece. The image is viewed on a monitor via an attached camera or with the naked eye. Light is transmitted from a remote light source through light cables that attach at the light guidepost. Fiber-optic light bundles pass through the insertion tube to the distal tip. Light cables may be steam sterilized for laparoscopy and cystoscopy, and most models can be immersed for disinfection (check with the manufacturer). Be sure that the light cables in your inventory attach securely to the telescope. Adapters are available for different models.

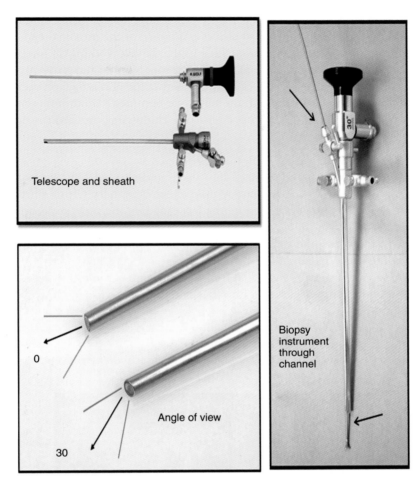

Figure 1.2 Rigid telescope.

Rigid telescopes differ in outer diameters, viewing angles, and lengths, depending on their use (shown in Figure 1.2). These differences make them a versatile endoscope, especially when used in conjunction with an operating sheath. The o.d. can range from 1 to 10 mm, with lengths ranging from 18 to 30 cm. The most common telescope used in veterinary medicine is 2.7 mm by 18 cm with a 25 or 30° viewing lens.

The viewing angle refers to the middle of the viewing field, shown in Figure 1.2. A 0° tip will allow for a frontward view, whereas an angled tip allows for an increased field of view by rotating the instrument. The angle of the tip can range from 10 to 120°.

Operating sheaths surround the rigid scope by attachment at the base of the eyepiece. Although the operating sheath will increase the outer diameter of the scope, it will also increase the telescope's versatility. Sheaths possess different functioning components. Fixed stopcocks positioned at the proximal end allow attachment for irrigation, or suction. Sheaths that have a working channel allow flexible instruments to pass beyond the telescope for biopsies and retrieval of foreign bodies. Levers on the stopcock control whether the port is opened or closed. When these features are utilized, the telescope becomes a multipurpose scope used to perform procedures such as cystoscopy, rhinoscopy, and arthroscopy.

Flexible Endoscopes

Flexible endoscopes are categorized into video and all-fiber-optic endoscopes. Fiber-optic endoscopes are commonly used in the veterinary setting since they are less expensive to operate, despite the fact they lack the superior technology of a video endoscope.

Video endoscopes offer greater image quality, resolution, and color. Incorporated in the distal tip behind the objective lens is a video chip that converts the image to a digital signal. This signal transmits through connection wires to the video processor. The image is sent to an image capturing device, monitor, printer, or computer.

Instead of a video chip, the all-fiber-optic fiberscope, seen in Figure 1.3, utilizes coherent fiber-optic bundles that transmit the image to the eyepiece. In order to view the image on a monitor, a camera must be attached at the eyepiece. Both

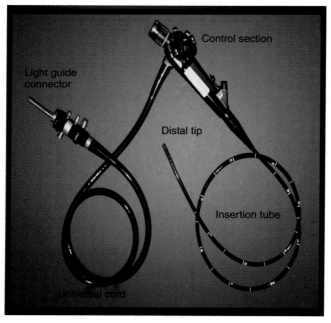

Figure 1.3 Basic flexible endoscope.

types of endoscopes utilize non-coherent fiber-optic bundles to transmit light to the distal tip for illumination.

The fibers are as thin as a human hair and are pliable. They are arranged in a bundle inside the endoscope and can bend in response to the endoscope's movements. Once these fibers come into contact with moisture, they become hard and brittle and can break, resulting in either a loss of light (non-coherent) or a loss of image (coherent). As a result, all ports are sealed to protect the interior from water intrusion.

There are wide varieties of endoscopes available in today's market. The o.d. can range from 2.5 to 11 mm and greater, with insertion tube lengths varying from 55 to 240 cm. Other mechanisms that will vary are a two- or four-way tip deflection, insufflation, aspiration, irrigation, and the size of the operating channel. When selecting an endoscope, it is important to understand the needs of the procedure and versatility of the endoscope, plus the length and outer diameter of the insertion tube of each endoscope. A small 2.5 mm o.d. by 100 cm endoscope can be utilized as a male cystoscope and a bronchoscope for a cat or toy-breed dog. A 5.3 mm by 100 cm pediatric gastroscope can double as a small toy-breed gastroscope or a bronchoscope for a large-breed dog. For the cat or small- to medium-sized dog (10–15 kg), a 7.8 mm o.d. × 100–110 cm scope would be adequate for an upper gastrointestinal procedure. In some medium- to large-sized dogs, this would only allow visualization just past the pylorus. If the same scope was 140 cm long, the duodenum would be obtainable for viewing and a more thorough evaluation could be accomplished. Table 1.1 gives examples of flexible endoscope sizes and procedures. The procedural chapters review and discuss the best endoscope(s) for a given procedure.

An endoscope with four-way deflection, aspiration, and air/ water capability is essential for performing a gastrointestinal procedure. The degree of deflection should be 90 to 100 in a left and right direction with 180 to 210 deflections up and down. A bronchoscope may only need a two-way deflection with angulations of 90 degrees whereas a cystoscope may have two-way deflection of 270 degrees.

Nomenclature

Whether video or fiber-optic, all flexible endoscopes have similar features. Proper endoscope handling, troubleshooting, and maintenance of the endoscope are accomplished when the inner workings of the endoscope are understood. There will be slight differences depending on the manufacturer, but for our purposes, a four-way gastroscope will be discussed.

The basic sections of a flexible endoscope (Figure 1.3) are the light guide connector or terminal end, universal or umbilical cord, control section, operating channel, insertion tube, bending section, and distal tip. Each section houses delicate internal structures.

Table 1.1 Examples of flexible endoscopes and their uses.

Use	2.5 mm × 55 cm/ 2-way deflection	3.8 mm × 55 cm/ 2-way deflection	5.0 mm × 55 cm/ 2-way deflection	5.3 mm × 100 cm/ 4-way deflection/ air/water	7.9-8.3 mm × 100-140 cm/ 4-way deflection/ air/water	11 mm × 240 cm/ 4-way deflection/ air/water
Cystoscopy/male dog	×					
Bronchoscopy/small breed and cat	×	×				
Bronchoscopy/large breed			×			
Nasalpharyngoscopy		×	×		×	
Esophagoscopy/gastroscopy			×		×	×
Duodenoscopy			×		×	×
Colonoscopy				×		×

Light guide connector

The light guide connector contains the light guide, air pipe, electronic contacts for a video system, water bottle connection, suction port, and pressure compensation valve. The light guide connector inserts into an external light source.

Umbilical cord

The umbilical cord connects the light guide connector to the control section. It houses the non-coherent fiber-optic bundles, air channel, water channel, and aspiration channel.

Control section

The control section houses the angulation control knobs, air/water and aspiration valves, operating channel port, and an eyepiece with a focus mechanism for the fiberscope, as shown in Figure 1.4. The angulation knobs, one for up and down and the other for left and right, control the deflection of the bending

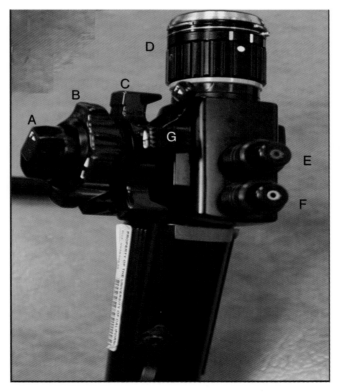

Figure 1.4 Control handle: A, locking device; B, knob that controls left and right movement of the distal tip; C, knob that controls up and down movement of the distal tip; D, eyepiece; E, suction valve; F, air/water valve; G, locking device.

section. Small wires travel from the knobs to a steel mesh at the distal part of the insertion tube. As the wires engage, the deflection occurs. The left thumb and right hand are used to manipulate the deflection knobs. Many endoscopes have a locking device associated with each knob that allows the endoscopist to maintain a desired degree of deflection while freeing up the right hand. Failure to disengage the locks can stretch control wires, causing them to snap, resulting in costly repairs.

The left first and second fingers manipulate the suction valve and the air/water valve, respectively. Air is introduced into the patient by lightly covering the top of the air/water valve. This forces air from the air/water bottle attached at the light guide through the insertion tube to the distal tip. Insufflation of the cavity will occur, which assists in visualization. Water is used to rinse the lens of debris – depressing the air/water valve completely will engage the air/water bottle to force water to the distal tip. The air/water system begins as two individual tubes that connect separately to the air/water valve. Depending on the manufacturer, the two may combine to become a common channel within the insertion tube or at the distal tip. Refer to the schematics in the manual when troubleshooting the air/water system.

Operating channel

The operating channel supports the suction and instrumentation function. A tube from the suction connector at the light guide travels through the umbilical cord connecting with the suction valve on the hand piece. From there, the tubing travels to the distal tip. The insertion tube is where the suction and biopsy share the operating channel. When the suction valve is depressed, the hole in the valve stem enters the channel, allowing external suction to pull fluids and air from the body cavity.

Flexible instruments are introduced into the operating channel at the instrument channel port. Biopsy and retrieval forceps are most common, but laser fibers can also be utilized.

Insertion tube

The insertion tube is the working end of the endoscope. It is composed of a hollow tube made from steel coil, fiber mesh, and vulcanized rubber. The outer layer is marked with metric measurements. It provides protection for the delicate internal components while maintaining the flexibility needed to maneuver within the body cavities, as shown in Figure 1.5b. Within the tube are the angulation wires, air/water channels, operating channel, non-coherent bundles, and coherent bundles or microchip connection wires, as shown in Figure 1.5a. Manipulating the insertion tip should be performed with caution. Over-torquing can

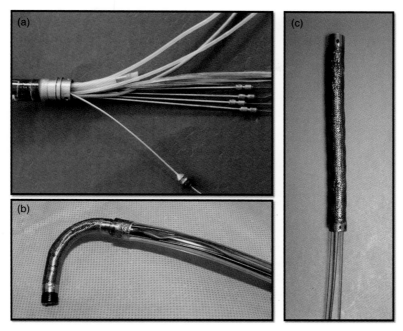

Figure 1.5 (a) Internal components of the insertion tube include deflection wires ×4, fiber-optic bundles, air/water channel, and biopsy/instrument channel. (b) Clear sheathed scope showing manipulation of internal components. (c) Bending section: flexible steel mesh holds the wires that travel from the control knobs to the bending section.

compromise fiber-optic bundles, which can lead a decrease in either illumination or visualization. The length and outer diameter of the insertion tube will vary depending on the function of the endoscope.

Bending section
This is where tip deflection occurs. The angulation wires (see Figure 1.5c) attach to the control knobs and act as a pulley system at the distal tip. There is one wire for each direction – up, down, left, and right. The degree of deflection should be monitored. Over time, the wires begin to stretch and may break, which can inhibit or prevent the endoscope from functioning properly during the diagnostic test performed.

Distal tip
At the end of the insertion tube is the distal tip, which is where the light guides, operating channel, and air/water nozzle terminate. The objective lens protects fiber-optic bundles or a video chip and is housed here. A complete diagram is shown in Figure 1.6.

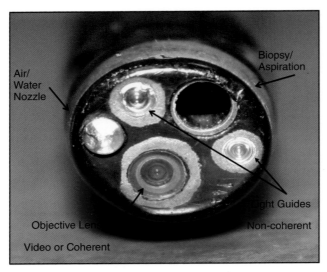

Figure 1.6 Distal tip. Light guides contain the non-coherent fibers and the objective lens houses coherent fibers or a video chip.

ANCILLARY EQUIPMENT

Instrumentation

A wide variety of instrumentation is available. The instrument diameter needs to be slightly smaller than the biopsy channel diameter. For example, an endoscope with a 2 mm channel will need a 1.8 mm o.d. instrument. Forceps larger than the biopsy channel can cause breaks or tears in the channel, which can lead to further internal damage and costly repairs. Forceps should also be at least 10 cm longer than the biopsy channel to allow the assistant to obtain diagnostic biopsy samples comfortably. Biopsy instruments are flexible forceps that pass through the operating channel of either rigid or flexible endoscopes. Variations can include spiked, cup, oval, fenestrated, serrated, or smooth. As the jaws are opened outside the endoscope, then closed onto the mucosa, a biopsy sample is taken. The forceps are removed and the sample is retrieved.

Cytology brushes and guarded microbiology brushes are used to obtain mucosal cytology/culture samples. Brushes are deployed to retrieve the sample, then pulled back into the casing to shield the sample from contamination.

Foreign body retrieval forceps are used to retrieve items such as bones, toys, or any other foreign material. Snares, baskets, rat tooth, two-prong, and Roth nets are some examples (shown in Figure 1.7). Chapter 4 outlines their usage, and additional equipment essential to a procedure is reviewed in later chapters.

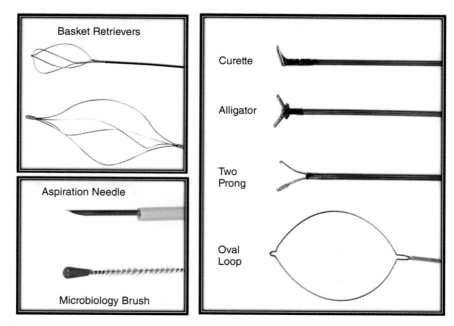

Figure 1.7 Instrumentation used for foreign body retrieval and cytology sampling.

Endoscope Components
Light source
A powerful light source is essential for the illumination of the mucosa. The quality of the video images obtained for patient documentation is dependent on the quality of the light produced. Light sources include 150 W halogen and 300 W xenon bulbs. LED light sources are also available. Xenon bulbs are recommended for video endoscopes. The xenon bulb produces more light, which creates better illumination. The quality of the light created produces a "white light" that is closer to natural light, and truer color of the tissue is observed. The light intensity of the halogen bulb is controlled manually. The xenon bulb can be controlled manually or automatically by the video processor and continuously adjusts for illumination and color. Most light sources have light guide adaptors to complement scopes made by different manufacturers. For smaller fiberscopes that do not require air/water capabilities, a portable battery-operated LED light source is available. It attaches to the light guidepost and eliminates the need for a large component. Further information on light sources in relation to laparoscopy can be found in Chapter 9.

Suction
A portable or in-house suction device is necessary for aspiration of air and fluids in a body cavity. Suction tubing is attached at the terminal end of flexible endoscopes or on the sheath of rigid telescopes.

Always make sure that the biopsy cap is closed before suctioning. Note that the hole in the suction valve is no larger than a grain of rice, so be wary of aspirating large particles that could plug the endoscope.

Monitor

The monitor is used for viewing the procedure. Cables attached from the camera or the video processor transport the image. High-definition (HD) monitors provide clear, precise images. A medical-grade monitor with full HD (1920 × 1080) resolution will provide an image with true color, brightness, and resolution. The monitor should include various video inputs a such as a 15-pin VGA computer input, two-way BNC composite video, Y/C, and HDMI video formats of 720, 1080I, and 1080P. It should also include video outputs for incorporation of image-capturing devices if needed. They come in various sizes from 19 to 55 in. Some models are also available with wireless features.

Monitors can be set for a "live feed," where just the image is seen, or be programmed to incorporate patient information through an attached keyboard. When images are captured, this information is also included. Comments such as image location can also be attached.

Image capture

A video endoscope has a control button on the hand piece that captures an image, or a foot pedal controlled by the endoscopist can be used. Some video processors incorporate an SD card. Other image-capturing systems are connected either from the camera attachment or to the video processor. Image-capturing devices permit documentation of the procedure. Images and video clips can be transferred to the patient record through a computer program or stored in another storage device.

Endoscopy tower

An endoscopy tower houses the equipment necessary to perform an endoscopic procedure. It includes a monitor, video processor, camera, insufflation device for laparoscopy, and image-capturing device. Towers can be stationary or mobile. A complete endoscopy station is shown in Figure 1.8 and is discussed further in Chapter 10.

Cables leading to and from the monitor, video processor, and so on can be confusing and difficult to troubleshoot, especially if a procedure is imminent and the image is lost. Labeling of cables at both ends (inputs) and on the components can help quickly pinpoint where a loose cable should be connected. Cable attachments should be checked periodically on mobile cart components that travel over rough or unstable surfaces.

Endoscopic procedures are less invasive, decrease hospital recovery times, and are utilized in internal medicine in addition to the surgical operating room. Multiple endoscopes can be used with one system allowing for greater versatility. New devices such as battery-powered light sources and wireless receiver systems

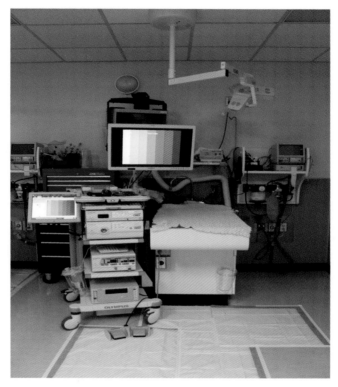

Figure 1.8 Work station with endoscopy tower.

are helping to transform endoscopy procedures performed outside the veterinary hospital. Endoscopes with HD technology have been recently introduced into the veterinary setting. Endoscopy continues to play a vital and important role in veterinary medicine.

SUGGESTED READING

McCarthy, T.C. (2005) *Veterinary Endoscopy for the Small Animal Practitioner*. Elsevier Saunders, St Louis, MO.
Riel, D.L. (2012) Care and maintenance of endoscopic equipment. Presented at the Spring Veterinary Symposium 2012.

RECOMMENDED WEBSITES

Endoscopy Support Services: http://www.endoscopy.com.
Karl Storz: http://www.karlstorz.com.
Olympus: http://www.olympusamerica.com.
Stryker: http://www.stryker.com.

2

Endoscope care and cleaning

Valerie Walker

William R. Pritchard Veterinary Medical Teaching Hospital, University of California-Davis, Davis, California, USA

Endoscopes are a costly investment for any veterinary practice. Owing to the delicate internal parts of flexible and rigid endoscopes, all clinical personnel who use and reprocess the equipment must have a basic understanding of how each endoscope functions and how to care for them appropriately. Knowledge of the working components and design of the endoscope is vital for proper cleaning and disinfection, troubleshooting problems, and extending the life of the endoscope.

To prevent infectious complications from flexible endoscopic procedures, it is critical to understand the importance of a proper cleaning protocol. Infections can arise from endogenous and exogenous microbes. Microbes from the gastrointestinal or respiratory tract can be introduced into the bloodstream or other sterile parts of the body from the endoscopic procedure. Exogenous infections can be transmitted from patient to patient from contaminated endoscopes or ancillary equipment, contaminated working surfaces, and improper cleaning and disinfecting protocols.

The Association for Professionals in Infection Control (APIC) created guidelines specific to the cleaning and high-level disinfection of endoscopes, which are endorsed by the American Society for Gastrointestinal Endoscopy and the Society of Gastrointestinal Nurses and Associates (SGNA).

COMPONENTS OF A COMPLETE CLEANING PROTOCOL

Each endoscope is unique, and the manufacturer's guidelines must be followed for care, cleaning, and disinfecting.

A non-abrasive, low-foaming enzymatic detergent should be used for cleaning the endoscope and accessories, followed by treatment with a high-level

Endoscopy for the Veterinary Technician, First Edition. Edited by Susan Cox.
© 2016 John Wiley & Sons, Inc. Published 2016 by John Wiley & Sons, Inc.

disinfectant (HLD) that is non-harmful to the rubber and metal components of the endoscope. Enzymatic detergent use is an important initial step in the endoscope cleaning protocol, as it can break down proteins from blood and tissue left within the channels. Without the use of an enzymatic solution, debris left behind from an endoscopic procedure and exposed to HLDs can become rock-hard and plug channels. Dilution and variations in water temperature when using an enzymatic cleaner can alter its effectiveness, so it is necessary to follow the manufacturer's guidelines.

An HLD is defined as a chemical germicide that is capable of destroying all viruses, vegetative bacteria, fungi, mycobacteria, and some but not all bacterial spores. HLDs are used to ensure the destruction of microorganisms in the internal channels and also the exterior of the endoscope.

The type of HLD used will be determined by the manufacturer's recommendations and type of reprocessing available (automatic endoscope reprocessor or manual). Automatic endoscope reprocessors reduce the exposure of personnel to chemical HLDs and provide a standardized cleaning routine.

Certain HLD products can cause functional and cosmetic damage to the endoscope. Endoscope manufacturers differ on which HLDs are compatible with their endoscopes, so check before use. HLD 30-day solutions containing surfactants may have a longer shelf life, but can leave a soapy residue that is difficult to remove when rinsing and should be avoided.

Some types of HLD available on the market today include 2.4% glutaraldehyde, 0.55% *ortho*-phthalaldehyde (OPA), accelerated hydrogen peroxide 2%, and 7.5% hydrogen peroxide with 0.23% peracetic acid. Personal protective attire, such as gloves and eyewear, should be worn when working with enzymatic cleaners and HLDs.

Once HLDs are activated, viability can vary with each product. Test strips, as shown in Figure 2.1, are available and should be used daily and logged. HLDs should be changed if the strip indicates, even if the solution's expiry date has not been reached.

Table 2.1 presents some common problems that may occur before, during and after an endoscopic procedure, and possible solutions that may be employed. This table can be consulted if any difficulties are encountered.

CLEANING PROTOCOLS

Endoscopes should be cleaned promptly after each procedure. Following the procedure at tableside, retest the suction, insufflation and water capabilities. The air/water channel should be flushed using the air/water cleaning valve (see examples in Figure 2.2) if available or, using the air/water valve, flush copious amounts of water, then air to rinse any debris in the channel. Suction water or enzymatic solution through the suction/biopsy channel. Alternating the tip in

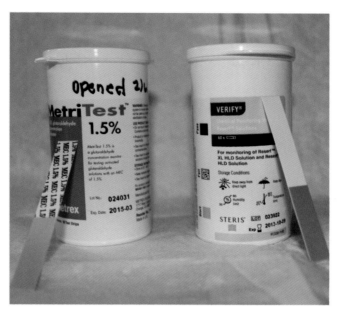

Figure 2.1 Two types of test strips to check HLD concentration. This step should be performed daily and the HLD replaced when strip indicates, regardless of whether the expiry date has been reached.

and out of the water while suctioning will help to agitate the debris loose from within the channels. Suctioning should continue until a clear stream of water can be seen in the suction hose attachment.

It is good practice to turn off all components before detaching the endoscope. Secure the scope at the working station and wipe down the insertion tube to remove debris. Place all safety caps over electronic ports as regulated by the manufacturer.

At this time, the endoscope should be moved to a designated cleaning station with a sink available. Using an enzymatic cleaning solution and a gauze pad, immerse and wipe the exterior of the endoscope, paying close attention to raised areas and control knobs. A soft-bristled toothbrush will help with removing debris from crevices. Gently brush the distal tip.

Leak Testing

Leak testing should be performed after every procedure and prior to immersing the endoscope to prevent fluid invasion repairs and to ensure the integrity of the scope, as discussed in Chapter 1. This will also eliminate potential cross-contamination. Leak testing can be accomplished with an automated constant air infuser or with a hand-held bulb and gauge device. Attach the leak tester to the venting connector. Place the distal tip including the bending section

Table 2.1   Troubleshooting.

Problem	Possible reason	Possible solution
No image transferred to monitor	Proper input channel selection	Select correct input
	All connecting components are turned on	Ensure all components into and out of monitor are turned on
	Proper attachment of video input and out-put cords	Ensure all attachments are secure
Image not centered on monitor	Camera attachment	Reattach the camera with proper alignment
Blurred image	Dirty eyepiece or camera adapter	Wipe with alcohol-moistened swab
	Dirty objective lens	Flush water across lens
	Out of focus	Use diopter on scope to focus or camera focus
	Distortion of colors	White balance
Hazy image/image stain	Water damage of internal parts	Send to manufacturer for repair
	Damaged objective lens	
	Rigid telescope	
	Damaged glass rod/lens system	
Image too intense	Light source settings	Adjust brightness control on light source
	Too close to mucosa	Back endoscope out to regain luminal view
Image too dark	Insertion of light guide or terminal end into light source	Firmly reinsert terminal end
	Light source settings	Adjust brightness control on light source
	Broken non-coherent fiber-optic bundles	Send to manufacturer for repair – kinking and tightly wrapping the scope can damage the fiber-optic bundles
	Halogen or xenon bulb	Ensure light source has been ignited Replace bulb
No image/black spots	Electrical problem	Send to manufacture for repair
	Broken coherent fiber-optic bundles	Kinking and tightly wrapping the scope can damage fiber-optic bundles or fluid invasion occurred when water and other fluids entered dry parts of the flexible scope, making fiber-optic bundles brittle
		Send to manufacturer for repair
No air	Air/water pump	Ensure unit is on
	Insertion of light guide or terminal end into light source	Firmly reinsert terminal end.
	Over-filled water bottle.	Remove water to fill level
	O-ring in water bottle	Inspect O-ring in water bottle cap, replace or change water bottle

Table 2.1 (*Continued*)

Problem	Possible reason	Possible solution
	Air/water valve skirt or O-ring.	Inspect valve and replace or change valve
		Inspect and clean valve, lubricate according to manufacturer's recommendations
	Dirty air/water valve	Inspect and clean
	Air/water exit nozzle	Soaking the tip in enzymatic solution can help soften debris prior to brushing
		Never attempt to remove debris with a sharp object
		Use reverse suction to remove debris plug
	Blocked air channel	Send to manufacturer for repair
Insufficient water	Air/water pump	Ensure unit is on
	Insertion of light guide or terminal end into light source	Firmly reinsert terminal end
	Over-filled water bottle.	Remove water to fill level
	O-ring in water bottle	Inspect O-ring in water bottle cap, replace or change water bottle.
	Air/water valve skirt or O-ring	Inspect valve and replace or change
	Dirty air/water valve	Inspect and clean valve, lubricate according to manufacturer's recommendations.
	Blocked water channel	Use reverse suction technique to remove blockage (Box 2.2)
		Send to manufacturer for repair
Insufficient suction	Biopsy port cover	Ensure cover is in closed position
	Ancillary suction unit	Turn power on, inspect for proper attachment of suction line
	Dirty suction valve	Inspect and clean valve
	Blocked channel	**If in use – remove from patient**
		Depress suction valve while alternating the distal tip in and out of a bowl water to dislodge blockage
		Flush water from the biopsy port to the distal tip
		Remove from light source, depress suction valve and flush from suction adapter to distal tip
		Brush suction/operation channel with cleaning brush and flush channel
		Use reverse suction technique to remove
		Send to manufacturer for repair if unable to remove blockage

(*continued*)

Table 2.1 (*Continued*)

Problem	Possible reason	Possible solution
No tip deflection	Deflection knobs in locked position.	Remove lock
	Deflection wire snapped or stretched	Send to manufacturer for repair. Angulation problems can be caused by over-torquing the bending portion of the scope. Fluid invasion can also damage the angulation system
Tip deflection reversed	Proper handling technique	Hold control section with left hand and allow insertion tube to hang or be supported straight. Test up/down and left/right deflection
Problems passing biopsy forceps	Instrument broken – wire snapped, bent coil, wings will not open	Test function of instrument prior to use. Check for burrs and protruding parts by rubbing a gloved hand or cotton ball over all surfaces of the accessory **NEVER** insert a malfunctioning instrument
	Endoscope in over-flexed or "J" position	Return endoscope to neutral position, pass forceps, reposition endoscope

Each endoscope has unique features: the guidelines in the user manual should be referred to and followed. If there are any questions, seek instructions from the manufacturer.

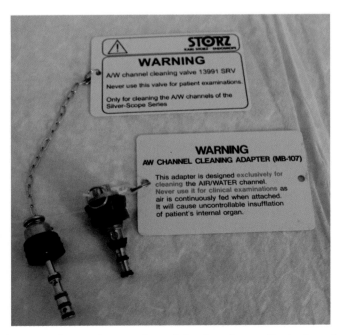

Figure 2.2 Olympus and Storz air/water channel cleaning adapters. Use in place of the air/water valve after the procedure is complete to flush water, then air, through all channels.

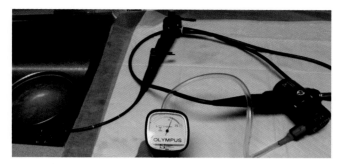

Figure 2.3 Leak testing a videoscope using a hand-held leak tester. The bending section is immersed to look for air bubbles at the A-rubber or from the distal tip, which is a sign of water invasion. Box 2.1 for complete guidelines.

in a bowl of enzymatic cleaner as shown in Figure 2.3. Engage the leak tester and watch for air bubbles. Deflecting the tip under the water can increase the success of finding smaller leaks. If a continuous flow of air bubbles is detected, or a continuous drop in pressure is visualized, stop the cleaning process and call the manufacturer. Full scope immersion is sometimes necessary to determine where the leak is originating from (do not immerse the leak tester). Step-by-step cleaning guidelines are given in Box 2.1.

BOX 2.1 ENDOSCOPE CLEANING GUIDELINES

A. *Pre-cleaning performed immediately post-procedure to remove gross debris*
  - With clean water, wipe down insertion tube
  - Aspirate water then air through suction channel until water aspirated is clear
  - Attach air/water channel cleaning valve (if available)
  - Flush water, then air, through channels
  - For endoscopes containing an elevator channel or auxiliary water channel – flush with water, then air
  - Disconnect from unit
  - Place water resistant cap to protect electrodes (videoscopes).
  - Move endoscope to reprocessing room
B. *Leak testing*
  - Inspect the leak tester
  - Attach the leak tester to the venting connector
  - Place the distal tip including the bending section in a bowl of enzymatic cleaner
  - Engage the leak tester and watch for air bubbles for 2 min
    - The A-rubber at the bending section will enlarge slightly; this is normal
    - If there is a leak at the bending section, deflecting the distal tip under water can increase the success of finding smaller leaks
    - Leaks from the biopsy channel will appear as bubbles emanating from the distal tip
    - Full endoscope immersion is sometimes necessary to determine where the leak is originating from

- If a continuous flow of air bubbles is detected, or a continuous drop in pressure is visualized, stop the cleaning process and call the manufacturer or repair center
- If a leak is detected and repairs must be made, the repair center may require you to continue the cleaning process to avoid cross-contamination
  - If no bubbles or drop in pressure are seen, release the pressure (hand-held) and leave attached to the endoscope for an additional 30 seconds, ensuring all air is removed

C. *Manual cleaning*
  - Remove all valves and biopsy port cover
  - Use a recommended enzymatic cleaner detergent solution
  - If using an endoscope tub, immerse the scope
  - Thoroughly wipe down all external surfaces. Use a soft brush to clean within the ridges of the control knobs and elevator channel opening if applicable. Clean the distal tip and remove any debris from the air/water nozzle
  - Insert the cleaning brush into the biopsy channel until it emerges from the distal tip. Clean the brush between insertions and repeat three times. If gross debris is still present, repeat until the brush emerges clean
  - Insert the cleaning brush into the suction valve port. Brush from the valve port towards the light guide connector until the brush emerges from the suction adaptor port. Repeat until clean
  - Insert the brush from the suction valve port towards the insertion tube until you reach the biopsy port. Repeat until clean
  - Insert a channel opening cleaning brush into the suction valve port and biopsy port. Care must be taken when inserting the brush into the air/water valve port. Debris can be pushed into the channel and an obstruction may occur, resulting in the need for repairs
  - Using clean enzymatic solution, attach the recommended suction cleaning adapter(s) and aspirate cleaning solution through all channels. Observe fluid streaming from all channels, including the air/water channel at the distal tip. If the air/water channel is clogged or a steady stream is not observed, Box 2.2
  - Repeat this process with clean water, then air, until fluid is removed from the endoscope. This prevents dilution or contamination of the HLD
  - Inspect and clean all valves and biopsy port

D. *High-level disinfecting*
  - Use a test strip or approved device to ensure the minimum recommended concentration specific to the product used
  - If using an automated endoscope reprocessing (AER) unit, attach appropriate connections. Start the unit as directed
  - If using a large basin or tub, leave the suction cleaning adaptor in place to aspirate the product into the channels
  - The duration of contact with the endoscope will vary. Read the label instructions for time and temperature variations
  - Rinse the endoscope with water and air. An AER unit will do this process
  - Flush with 70% isopropyl alcohol to assist the drying process
  - Hang the scope vertically to dry
  - Place the valves on a clean surface to air dry

If a leak is detected and repairs must be made, the repair center may require you to continue the cleaning process to avoid cross-contamination. Cleaning may be continued with constant pressure from the automated leak tester. Contact the repair technicians for further instructions. Continuation of the cleaning process may result in more damage to the interior of the scope and could result in a higher repair bill.

Brushing and Flushing (Figures 2.4–2.7)

If no leaks are detected, continue with the cleaning process. Flush the biopsy channel with enzymatic cleaner and brush all accessible channels with a cleaning brush of appropriate size. Clean the brush as it exits the endoscope to avoid recontaminating the channel. Endoscopes when purchased should come with a water bottle, channel brushes and the appropriate cleaning adapters. Brushes with bristles on both ends are available. Disposable, single-use brushes can also be purchased. Make sure the brush is of the appropriate size and in good condition, which ensures that all surfaces of the channel come into contact with the brush. Be aware that some endoscopes may have different sized brushes – the suction channel brush may be of a larger diameter than the biopsy channel brush. Brush the suction/instrument channel from the suction valve and out of the distal tip (the brush may need to be angled slightly), then from the suction valve to the suction connector through the umbilical tube. Lastly, use a short brush to clean

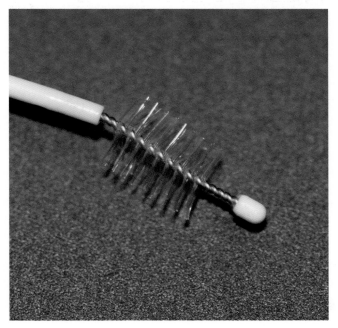

Figure 2.4 Bristled end of disposable channel cleaning brush. Note the blunt, rounded tip and fully intact bristles made to contact all areas of the channel. Brushes should be inspected before insertion into the endoscope.

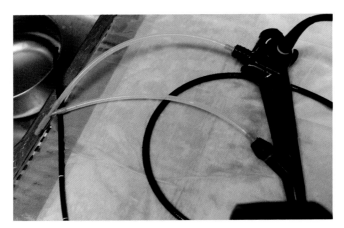

Figure 2.5 Cleaning/disinfection tubing adapter for a video bronchoscope – attaches to the suction port and biopsy port and allows flushing of enzymatic solution and HLD through the instrument/biopsy channel.

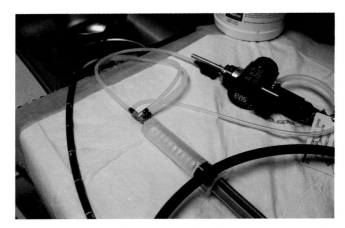

Figure 2.6 Cleaning adapter attached to the terminal end of a gastroscope. Various types of attachments are used for manual flushing and high-level disinfection. Included as a set are air pipe tubing, water bottle plug, suction port tubing, and tubing with a syringe adapter to flush all channels. See Figure 2.7 for adapters for the control section.

the biopsy port housing. Rinse the brush between insertions and repeat three times or more until the brush comes out clean. Attach all channel irrigation tubing to the appropriate channels and flush with copious amounts of enzymatic solution.

The air/water channel and the nozzle at the distal tip (see Figure 1.6) is too small to accommodate a cleaning brush, and can easily become clogged with debris. See Box 2.2 for guidelines if the air/water channel is compromised. Rinse

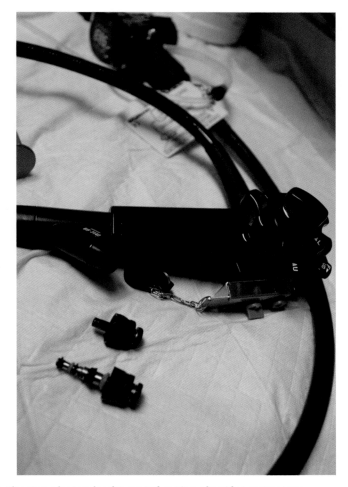

Figure 2.7 Cleaning adapters for the control section of a video gastroscope.

with water and flush air through the channels to remove excess fluid to avoid dilution of the HLD solution (see Figure 2.8). The endoscope must be thoroughly cleaned prior to immersion into an HLD.

Disinfection

Automated endoscopy processors (AERs), such as the model shown in Figure 2.9, are available for high-level disinfection. They reduce the risk of exposure from HLDs, provide consistent irrigation of chemical agents though all channels, and provide controlled soaking times. A large immersion bin, pictured in Figure 2.10, in a well-ventilated area is most widely used in veterinary medicine. The bin should be large enough to accommodate a loosely coiled scope. Owing to the fragile nature of the fiber-optics, an endoscope should never be coiled less than

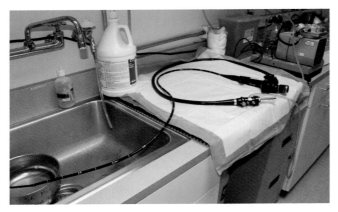

Figure 2.8 Reverse flushing a gastroscope. Box 2.2 for guidelines.

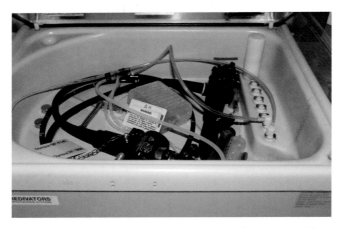

Figure 2.9 An endoscope ready for processing in an automated reprocessor. These types of units save time and reduce exposure to HLDs. To hold small objects such as valves or brushes, a mesh bag or plastic soap holder with perforations may be used.

12 in. Submerse the scope in an HLD such as a 2.4% alkaline solution of glutaraldehyde. Use the all-channel irrigation system to flush solution through all ports. A minimum soaking time of 20 min at 20 °C (room temperature) is necessary to ensure that high-level disinfection has occurred.

Rinse the endoscope thoroughly with copious amounts of water to remove the HLD solution from all channels. Flush with 70% alcohol, then air, and apply forced air if available to aid the drying process. The endoscope should be hung vertically with all ports open to facilitate drying and prevent microbial growth.

Valves should be cleaned with the same enzymatic solution using a soft brush and pipe cleaners for small holes on the valve stem. Depress suction valves to expose the hole, as shown in Figure 2.11. Valves should be exposed to the same

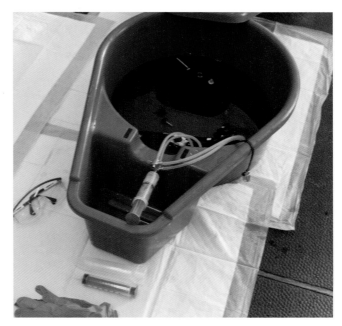

Figure 2.10 An endoscope inside an immersion bin. Enzymatic solution, then HLD solution, is aspirated through a syringe attached to the endoscope's all-channel irrigation tubing.

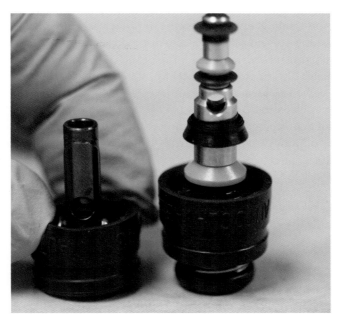

Figure 2.11 Examples of suction and air/water valves. The suction valve must be depressed to expose the hole for thorough cleaning. Rubber O-rings should also be inspected for tears.

HLD as the endoscope for the appropriate time period. During the cleaning process, the O-rings should be inspected for tears. High-level disinfection is also recommended for cleaning brushes and any other ancillary equipment (mouth gags, dental mirrors, etc.) that are reused.

Coil-wrapped wire retrieval or biopsy forceps should be immersed in enzymatic solution and wiped down after use. A small brush should be applied gently on the working end to remove gross debris. Ultrasonic cleaning is then recommended for 30–45 min using enzymatic solution, then water. The forceps should be hung to dry overnight, then packaged for steam sterilization.

ENDOSCOPE HANDLING BEFORE AND AFTER THE PROCEDURE

Owing to the delicate internal parts of flexible and rigid endoscopes, all personnel involved must have a basic understanding of how each endoscope functions and how to handle and care for them appropriately.

A routine inspection of the endoscope components pre- and post-procedure helps to reduce repair costs, ensures that equipment is well maintained for safe patient care, and extends the life of the endoscope.

Pre-procedure, inspect the exterior for any abnormalities such as dents, obvious punctures, or cracked lenses at the distal tip. Attach the endoscope to the appropriate system and attach a water bottle and suction tubing to appropriate ports at the terminal end. Depress the air/water valve to ensure a strong jet stream of water is rinsing the lens at the distal tip. Place the distal tip in a bowl of water and lightly cover the hole on top of the air/water valve. Observe sufficient air bubbles coming from the distal tip. While the tip is still submerged, test the suction valve for adequate fluid uptake. If the endoscope is not producing adequate air bubbles and/or does not have a strong water steam, there may be a small piece of debris plugging the channel. You must troubleshoot this problem before continuing the endoscopic procedure. For troubleshooting, see Box 2.2 for unblocking channel guidelines.

BOX 2.2 UNBLOCKING THE AIR/WATER CHANNEL – REVERSE FLUSHING

Blockage is determined to be in the air/water channel. The goal is to remove plugged debris from the small air/water channel. Suctioning enzymatic cleaning solution from the smaller distal tip to the larger diameter water bottle attachment port offers a greater chance of unplugging the channel.

- Supplies
  - Suction unit with attached tubing
  - Bowl of enzymatic cleaning solution in sink
  - Air/water valve attached

- ○ Closed-end tubing
- ○ Biopsy port cover attached and closed
- Procedure
  - ○ Distal tip in enzymatic solution
  - ○ Sealed/closed end tubing over air pipe at terminal end
  - ○ Insert suction unit tubing snugly into water bottle attachment port
  - ○ Turn on suction unit
  - ○ Depress air/water valve
  - ○ Watch for fluid in suction tubing
  - ○ Amount of fluid suctioned should increase as debris is removed.
  - ○ Continue for 1–2 min
  - ○ Detach from suction unit
  - ○ Plug endoscope into processor; attach water bottle and turn on component with air insufflation
  - ○ Depress air/water valve
  - ○ Observe sideways stream from distal tip
  - ○ May need to repeat if weak/no stream
  - ○ Other alternatives:
    - ■ Soak distal tip in warm enzymatic solution for 5–10 minutes, then reverse flush
    - ■ Suction hydrogen peroxide into the channel; allow to sit for 5 min, then reverse flush
- If the channel still blocked despite several reverse flush attempts, send the endoscope to an authorized repair center

Check the angulation of the tip deflection in each direction. Over time, the angulation wires may stretch or snap, resulting in costly repairs. White balancing of the endoscope should also be carried out prior to each procedure, as shown in Figure 2.12. This maneuver balances the color white between the endoscope

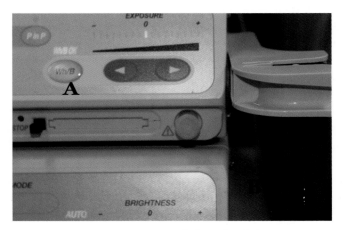

Figure 2.12 White balance. Some components include a white balance cup (B), or any white surface can be used. Insert the distal tip in the cup and depress the button (A), located on the video processor or camera box.

and the processor, allowing for a truer color image and picture. If any of these basic functions are not working, refer to Table 2.1 or the manufacturer's manual for troubleshooting tips prior to using the endoscope. Do not start a procedure with a malfunctioning endoscope.

Post-procedure tasks should include retesting of suction and air/water capabilities at the table side. A post-procedure check will help evaluate when or if a problem has occurred, pinpoint troubleshooting, and loosen gross debris from the endoscope prior to cleaning. If the endoscope is allowed to sit too long, it could cause a blockage in the air/water channel. See Box 2.2 for a complete checklist.

Cleaning Ancillary Equipment

Care must be taken to ensure the integrity of the endoscope and ancillary equipment. Everyone involved with using and maintaining endoscopy equipment should follow the same guidelines for proper handling.

The distal tip and light guide should be controlled at all times during transferring and operation of the endoscope. Dropping the tip against a hard surface can lead to damage to the objective lens or fiber-optic bundles, or could bend the air/water nozzle.

Kinking, over-twisting or torqueing of the umbilical cord or insertion tube could result in internal damage to the fiber-optic bundles and reduce the transfer of light through the non-coherent bundles or image transfer to the eyepiece through coherent bundles. It could also jeopardize the integrity of the operating channel. Passage of instrumentation could become difficult and small rents in the channel could occur. This could lead to costly repairs due to internal fluid leakage.

Sharp objects such as dental probes or needles should not be allowed near the endoscope. Small punctures could result in internal water damage. Mouth speculae should always be in place during a procedure to prevent damage to the endoscope.

Proper functioning of accessory instrumentation such as biopsy forceps or foreign body retrieval forceps should always be checked prior to insertion. If insertion of the instrument is difficult and the endoscope is in a flexed position, straighten the endoscope and try again. Never force any instrument through the operating channel.

Camera attachments and video processor adaptor cords should be evaluated for damage. The electronic prongs and pins used in these attachments should be free of debris and oxidation, and kept dry. Avoid damage to the internal wires by coiling the cord properly when storing and being aware of chairs, equipment, and personnel rolling or stepping on the cords during or after a procedure.

Light cables used for rigid and small-diameter flexible endoscopes should be inspected for small punctures and leakage of light. If leaks are detected, the fiber-optic bundles can become hard and brittle due to water damage through immersion or sterilization, thus decreasing the light transmission ability of the cable. Decreased light transmission can also be caused by over-bending or direct impact. Proper storage and correct sizing of sterilization pouches are important.

Light sources house either halogen or xenon bulbs. It is important to become familiar with the lamp housing to be able to change the bulb quickly when failure occurs. Most video processors switch to a back-up halogen bulb within the unit. Owing to the expense and limited shelf life of the xenon bulb, it is more economical to have a back-up halogen bulb on hand. This will allow for continuation of the endoscope procedure and allow overnight shipping of a new xenon bulb.

Well maintained equipment will decrease the frequency of damage and reduce repair costs, and will also result in safer patient care. It is important to read the equipment manual designated for your endoscope. The manual will specify trouble-shooting, how to clean the endoscope, and what cleaning and HLD products are safe and approved for use.

Storing Endoscopes

Endoscopes should be stored vertically and safely, ideally in an area away from excessive traffic. Endoscopes stored in their cases can be a reservoir for bacterial growth, especially if not thoroughly dried (ultrathin cystoscopes are an exception due to their delicate nature, so thorough drying before storage is essential). Valves and electrode caps can remain detached to ensure that the drying process is complete. Suggestions for endoscope storage can be found in Chapter 11.

Endoscope cases should be kept in the event that the endoscope needs to be sent for repair. Most endoscopes come with a pressure compensation cap in the event of ethylene oxide sterilization or shipping. This cap equalizes the pressure within the endoscope and attaches at the same port as the leak tester. Check with the delivery carrier – most airplanes have pressurized baggage compartments, and the ETO cap may not be necessary. Make sure that the endoscope is fully within the case – insertion tubes can easily be crushed when the case is closed. Most repair centers require a repair form enclosed with the endoscope. These are usually found on the repair center's website.

ENDOSCOPE DOCUMENTATION

A log containing information such as procedure, endoscopist and assistant, instrumentation used, ease of procedure, problems with procedure and equipment, pre-procedure check/post-procedure check, and cleaned/HLD will help pinpoint when an occurrence happened, troubleshoot repeated repair problems, and help others to learn how to use the equipment properly. This is especially helpful if equipment is shared between services.

CONCLUSION

The number of people handling an endoscope affects its lifetime. The higher the number of staff members handling an endoscope equates to more frequent repairs. Endoscopy units with a dedicated reprocessing staff have fewer repairs than those units where the staff-at-large is responsible for reprocessing. Following the guidelines and recommendations from the endoscope manufacturer, having proper cleaning protocols in place, knowledge of the intricate working parts, proper handling skills, and the ability to troubleshoot problems will reduce repair costs and extend the life of the endoscope.

SUGGESTED READING

Day, M.E. (Chair) (2012) *Standards of Infection Control in Reprocessing of Flexible Gastrointestinal Endoscopes.* SGNA Practice Committee, Chicago, IL, revised 2012.

Radlinski, M.G. (ed.) (2009) Endoscopy. *Vet. Clin. North Am. Small Anim. Pract.,* **39**(**5**), 817–992.

Riel, D.L. (2012) Care and maintenance of endoscopic equipment. Presented at the Spring Veterinary Symposium 2012.

Rutala, W.A. and APIC Guidelines Committee (1996) APIC guideline for selection and use of disinfectants. *Am. J. Infect. Control,* **24**(**4**), 313–342.

Tams, T.R. and Rawlings, C.A (eds) (2011) *Small Animal Endoscopy,* 3rd edn. Elsevier Mosby, St Louis, MO.

RECOMMENDED WEBSITES

Endoscopy Support Services: http://www.endoscopy.com.

Karl Storz: http://www.karlstorz.com.

Olympus: http://www.olympusamerica.com.

Stryker: http://www.stryker.com.

3 Anesthesia considerations for the endoscopy patient

Jody Nugent-Deal

William R. Pritchard Veterinary Medical Teaching Hospital, University of California-Davis, Davis, California, USA

Veterinary technicians are often called upon to anesthetize patients for diagnostic and surgical endoscopic procedures. In addition to the endoscopic procedures discussed in the following chapters, minimally invasive surgery such as laparoscopy and one-lung ventilation techniques using endoscopic equipment are also becoming more commonplace in veterinary medicine. Anesthetizing patients for these types of procedures can be challenging, so it is important to review basic techniques, and also to be exposed to more advanced methods should they be required. The scope of this chapter is focused on providing quality anesthesia for canine and feline patients undergoing endoscopy outlined in the following chapters.

DESIGNING AN ANESTHETIC PROTOCOL

Although the veterinary technician does not make the ultimate decision when choosing an anesthetic protocol, it is still important to understand how specific drugs work and why they are chosen for each individual patient. A thorough physical examination and baseline blood work should be evaluated prior to choosing an anesthetic protocol. Baseline blood work may be as simple as a packed cell volume (PCV), total protein (TP), blood glucose (BG), and AZO stick. This is the minimum suggested for healthy patients under the age of 7 years. For patients with underlying diseases or those over the age of 7 years, a complete blood count (CBC), biochemistry panel, and urinalysis (UA) should be evaluated. Other diagnostics such as radiographs, ultrasound, and specific blood tests may be considered based on the patient and the presenting complaint(s).

Each anesthetic protocol should be tailored to fit the needs of the individual patient. Current physical examination findings, blood work and diagnostic test results, age, species, disease status, previous medical/surgical history, and any previous anesthetic complications are taken into account. The anesthetist should take into consideration the anticipated problems for each patient undergoing anesthesia. Anticipated problems for any patient under anesthesia include hypothermia, hypoventilation, hypotension, and bradycardia. Why are these anticipated problems for all patients under anesthesia? These are potential negative side-effects caused by the anesthetic drugs that are administered. Hypothermia can be caused by vasodilation, an open body cavity, and the lack of temperature regulation under anesthesia. Bradycardia and hypoventilation are generally direct effects of opioid administration. Inhalant anesthetics cause dose-dependent vasodilation that can lead to hypotension. Anesthetists should be aware of these potential side-effects and how they are treated.

There are potential additional anticipated problems for anesthetic patients, which are based on the physical examination findings, diagnostic results, disease status, and procedure being performed. Examples of additional anticipated problems include, but are not limited to: blood loss, anemia, arrhythmias, airway obstruction, hypertension, hypo- or hyperglycemia, and slow drug metabolism. The individual patient should be assessed prior to making a final anesthetic plan. Box 3.1 provides a list of anesthetic considerations for any procedure.

BOX 3.1 GENERAL CONSIDERATIONS FOR ANY ANESTHETIZED PATIENT

- Unless contraindicated, premedications should be administered
- All patients should have an IV catheter placed prior to anesthetic induction
- All patients should be intubated during the procedure regardless of time under anesthesia
- Management of hypotension in any of these patients is generally maintained by decreasing the percentage of inhalant, fluid boluses of a crystalloid or colloid (when safe), and the use of a positive inotrope (when appropriate)
- General fluid therapy is given at 5–10 mL/kg/h unless contraindicated
- At the minimum, basic monitoring equipment is used regardless of time under anesthesia (HR, RR and depth, CRT, MM color, pulse quality, jaw tone, eye position, temperature, blood pressure, heat support)
  - Advanced monitoring should be used when indicated – ECG, $ETCO_2$, SpO_2, ABG, etc.
- Post-operative pain management should be used when needed

reproduced with permission from Seymour, C. and Duke-Novakovski, T. (eds), *BSAVA Manual of Canine and Feline Anaesthesia and Analgesia*, 2nd edn, 2007. © BSAVA.

The American Society of Anesthesiologists (ASA) has formulated a status classification system (Table 3.1) which should be assigned to each patient prior to anesthetic drug administration. This system is used to categorize potential risks for the individual patient. Animals with a higher ASA status are considered to be at a greater risk for anesthetic complications. These patients generally require multiparameter monitoring to improve their chances of a successful recovery.

Table 3.1   ASA Physical Status Classification System.

Classification	Definition
ASA Physical Status 1	A normal healthy patient
ASA Physical Status 2	A patient with mild systemic disease
ASA Physical Status 3	A patient with severe systemic disease
ASA Physical Status 4	A patient with severe systemic disease that is a constant threat to life
ASA Physical Status 5	A moribund patient who is not expected to survive without the operation

Source: based on the Physical Status Classification System of the American Society of Anesthesiologists, Park Ridge, IL, USA; www.asahq.org.

Goals of Premedication and Sedation: Why are Premedications So Important?

Providing patients with a premedication can make catheter placement and anesthetic induction less stressful for both the anesthetist and the patient. Premedicating the patient can also help facilitate handling and restraint, which in turn increases safety. Lastly, many premedications not only provide analgesia and sedation, but also contribute to a "balanced" or "multimodal" technique that can reduce the overall amount of drugs needed for anesthetic induction and maintenance.

Ideal properties of premedication and sedation drugs should include the following:

• produce sedation and analgesia
• have minimal effects on the cardiovascular system
• have minimal effects on the liver and kidneys
• cause minimal respiratory depression
• have the ability to reverse the drug
• inexpensive

Unfortunately there is no single drug that possesses all of these characteristics; therefore, we must carefully choose a combination of drugs to obtain the desired effects we are looking for. When appropriate combinations of drugs are used in conjunction with each other, it often allows for overall lower doses to be administered. Many drug combinations work synergistically with each other. Common drug combinations include α_2-agonists given with opioids and phenothiazines such as acepromazine given with opioids (neuroleptanalgesia). Opioids combined with midazolam and/or acepromazine is also another common drug combination.

Common routes of administration include intravenous, intramuscular, subcutaneous, and oral. The route of administration can greatly affect the time to peak effect and the bioavailability of the drug. This will vary by drug, hence a formulary should be consulted prior to administration.

Monitoring Equipment

One of the best pieces of monitoring equipment is an experienced anesthetist! While it is obviously important to monitor blood pressure, oxygenation, and so on, it is equally important also to monitor the patient visually. The anesthetist should regularly monitor palpebral reflex, toe pinch, jaw tone, heart and respiratory rates, depth of the breath, capillary refill time, and mucus membrane color.

Monitoring a patient's vital signs under general anesthesia is extremely important. The extent of monitoring will depend on the ASA status of the patient and the procedure being performed. At a minimum, the heart rate, respiratory rate, pulse quality, mucus membrane color and capillary refill time, core body temperature, and blood pressure should be monitored continuously and recorded onto an anesthetic record every 5 min. Additional monitoring can include electrocardiography, capnography, pulse oximetry, arterial blood gas monitoring, direct arterial blood pressure, and central venous pressure monitoring. It is important to remember that anesthetic drugs can cause respiratory and cardiovascular depression in any patient regardless of age or disease status, hence anesthetic monitoring is mandatory.

There are many multiparameter anesthetic monitors on the market today, such as that shown in Figure 3.1. A multiparameter monitor generally has all or almost all of the common monitoring devices in one machine. Although these machines often make monitoring anesthesia more convenient, they are not necessary if you have access to individual pieces of equipment that can be used to meet the needs of each patient.

Blood Pressure Monitoring

Blood pressure should be monitored in any patient undergoing general anesthesia. It is important to maintain normotension during the anesthetic period. Normal blood pressure helps ensure adequate tissue perfusion of the major organs. Untreated hypotension can lead to organ damage or failure, shock, or even death. Blood pressure can be obtained using either direct (invasive) or indirect (non-invasive) methods. Non-invasive blood pressure monitoring (NIBP) is most commonly utilized and can be accomplished using either the oscillometric or Doppler method.

The Doppler method works by placing an ultrasonic probe over an artery. With proper placement, the "whooshing" sound of the heart should be audible. A blood pressure cuff is then placed proximal to the probe, as shown in Figure 3.2. The cuff is occluded using a sphygmomanometer until the sound of the heart in no longer apparent. The cuff is then slowly deflated until the heart sounds return.

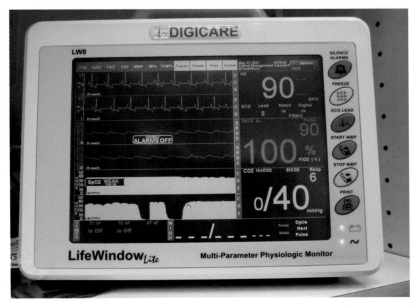

Figure 3.1 Multiparameter monitors allow the anesthetist to monitor multiple vital signs via one streamlined machine. Basic monitors include SpO_2, $ETCO_2$, NIBP, ECG, HR, RR, and temperature. More advanced models often include direct arterial blood pressure, gas analyzers, tidal volume, peak inspiratory pressure, and central venous pressure.

The first heart sound is considered the patient's systolic blood pressure. This is an easy and accurate way to obtain systolic blood pressure in both dogs and cats. This method also works well with smaller patients or those with short, stubby legs. Common sites used for Doppler probe placement include the metacarpal, metatarsal, and coccygeal arteries. Ideally, the chosen area should be free of hair. Ultrasound gel between the skin and the probe will make the heart sounds audible.

The oscillometric method uses a machine (Cardell®, petMAP®, Dinamap®) to calculate the heart rate and systolic, diastolic, and mean arterial blood pressure. Machines can be programmed to check the blood pressure at specific time intervals. Oscillometric methods can give inaccurate readings. This is most often experienced in patients that have arrhythmias, severe hypotension, or vasoconstriction, or those weighing less than 5 kg.

Cuff size is important regardless of what indirect method is chosen. In canine patients, the width of the cuff should extend about 40% of the circumference of the limb or tail. In the feline patient, the cuff should extend about 30–40%.

Direct blood pressure is considered the "gold standard" technique, as demonstrated in Figure 3.3. It is the only method that will give continuous, real-time monitoring and it is the most accurate. Direct blood pressure monitoring does require specialized equipment and advanced training to catheterize the artery

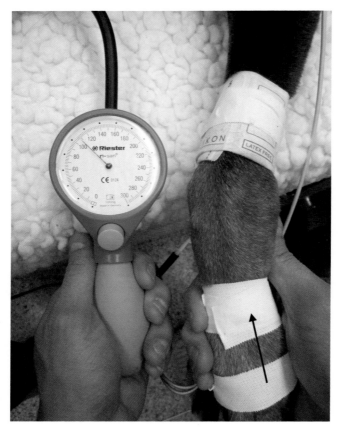

Figure 3.2 NIBP can be monitored using either a Doppler probe and sphygmomanometer (as illustrated) or an oscillometric unit. The Doppler probe gives only systolic blood pressure, but is considered to be more accurate in most patients than other NIBP methods. The Doppler probe is placed over the artery distal to the large carpal foot pad. The arrow indicates approximate probe placement on the leg (the probe is actually located on the palmar surface).

and maintain patency properly. Invasive blood pressure monitoring is suggested for patients that are critically ill or at an increased risk for complications. The arteries used for cannulation in the dog include the dorsal pedal, auricular, coccygeal, femoral, and palmar, with the dorsal pedal artery being the most common. The dorsal pedal and coccygeal arteries are most commonly used in the feline patient. Regardless of species, the dorsal pedal artery is the easiest for maintaining postoperatively.

Hypotension

Regardless of how blood pressure is monitored, hypotension should be treated when present. Hypotension can be treated in several ways. In general, the first

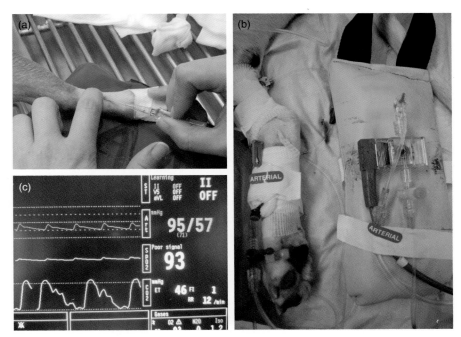

Figure 3.3 Direct arterial blood pressure monitoring gives a continuous, real-time reading of systolic, mean, and diastolic blood pressure. This method is considered the "gold standard." (a) The artery is first cannulated with a standard catheter. (b) A transducer is attached to both the catheter and the monitor. Source: photo courtesy of Dr. Cary Craig, Clinical Professor Small Animal Anesthesia, UC Davis Veterinary Medical Teaching Hospital. (c) The monitor shows continuous and real-time readings of the blood pressure.

step is to decrease the vaporizer setting if possible. If this does not work or if the inhalant cannot be reduced, the patient can be administered a 10–20 mL/kg bolus of crystalloid fluids (if safe for the patient). Crystalloids do not stay in the vascular space for long periods of time and an increase in blood pressure may be short lived.

Colloids are also another option for the treatment of hypotension. Colloids contain high molecular weight substances that stay within the vascular space for longer periods than crystalloids. Colloids are often used as a bolus starting with 5 mL/kg. If other treatment options are not possible or have failed, positive inotropes can be employed and are administered as a constant-rate infusion.

Capnography

Capnography provides a non-invasive method for measuring end-tidal carbon dioxide ($ETCO_2$). Capnometry is the numerical display of $ETCO_2$. The capnogram is the graphical display of $ETCO_2$ and capnography or the capnograph is the technique or instrument used to measure $ETCO_2$. In many cases, people use the term capnography as an all-inclusive term for all of the above.

$ETCO_2$ is the expired amount of carbon dioxide exhaled from the patient. Normal $ETCO_2$ levels range between 35 and 45 mmHg in most mammals. Patients are considered hypercapnic (too much CO_2) when $ETCO_2$ is greater than 45 mmHg. Increased values indicate inadequate ventilation, rebreathing of CO_2, or hypoventilation. Prolonged values reading above 60 mmHg can lead to hypoxemia. Hypoxemia predisposes patients to arrhythmias, myocardial depression, respiratory acidosis, and, in rare cases, heart failure. In these cases, patients should be manually or mechanically ventilated to decrease $ETCO_2$. Hypoventilation can also indicate too deep an anesthetic plane. Vitals and depth should be assessed and anesthetic depth adjusted as needed.

$ETCO_2$ values that are less than 35 mmHg can indicate hyperventilation. These patients are considered hypocapnic (insufficient CO_2). Ventilation may also be required to help regulate erratic breathing patterns such as tachypnea. Hyperventilation can also indicate a light anesthetic plane or pain. This should obviously be assessed and dealt with accordingly. Hypocapnia can also indicate other issues such as V/Q mismatch, decreased cardiac output, esophageal intubation, extubation of the patient, kink or mucus plug in the tube, apnea, and hypothermia.

There are two types of capnographs on the market: sidestream and mainstream. Sidestream capnography requires a sample line to be connected directly to the airway, as shown in Figure 3.4b. This method offers continuous sampling by pumping gases through tubing into the measurement chamber. This is very effective but does have a higher chance of becoming kinked or clogged with blood, mucus, or moisture.

Mainstream capnography analyzes gas directly at the endotracheal tube where the device is attached, as shown in Figure 3.4a. The mainstream device can increase dead space, so it is important to use a pediatric piece when working with small patients. Mainstream monitors are less likely to become clogged and are often cheaper to maintain. The disadvantages are that they are larger than sidestream monitors and can pull or kink the endotracheal tube.

Electrocardiography

The electrocardiograph (ECG) is the only piece of equipment that will monitor both heart rate and rhythm. The ECG works by displaying a graphical representation of electrical activity in the heart. All mammals have a four-chambered heart. The initial electrical impulse starts in the sinoatrial (SA) node (the heart's natural pacemaker) located in the right atrium and then travels to the atrioventricular (AV) node located between the atria and the ventricles. The electrical impulse then travels through the Purkinje fibers and out through the ventricles. These electrical impulses produce the P-wave, QRS complex, and T-wave seen on the normal ECG.

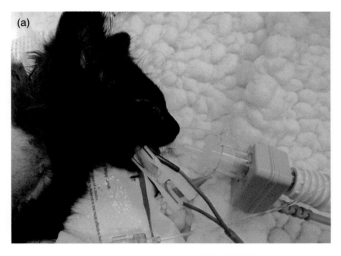

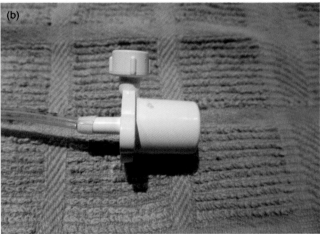

Figure 3.4 (a) Mainstream capnography analyzes gas directly at the endotracheal tube where the device is attached. The mainstream device can increase dead space so it is important to use a pediatric piece when working with small patients. Mainstream monitors are less likely to become clogged and are often cheaper to maintain. However, they are larger than sidestream monitors and can pull or kink the endotracheal tube. (b) Sidestream capnography requires a sample line to be connected directly to the airway. This method offers continuous sampling by pumping gases through tubing into the measurement chamber. This is very effective but does have a higher chance of becoming kinked or clogged with blood, mucus, or moisture.

The P-wave represents atrial depolarization. This occurs during contraction when blood is pumped from the atria into the ventricles. The QRS complex represents ventricular depolarization. This occurs when blood leaves the heart and travels to the lungs from the right ventricle or the rest of the body from the left ventricle. The T-wave represents ventricular repolarization. This occurs during relaxation when passive refilling of the ventricles takes place.

In veterinary medicine, the most common ECG used for monitoring under anesthesia is the three-lead system. There are various color schemes used for each lead, but most commonly a white lead is used for the right forelimb, a black lead for the left forelimb, and a red lead for the left hind limb. These leads can be placed on the animal using an ECG sticky pad attached to either the foot or chest/abdominal wall. Alligator clips can also be used, but the teeth should be flattened out when possible to help prevent trauma.

Pulse Oximetry

Pulse oximetry monitoring allows for non-invasive measurements of oxygen saturation of arterial hemoglobin. Common sites for probe placement include the pinna, foot, prepuce, vulva, lip, tongue, or anywhere there is a non-pigmented area of skin. Heavily furred and pigmented areas can affect the monitor's accuracy. Vasoconstriction, hypovolemic shock, dry mucus membranes, hypothermia, interference with ambient light, motion/shivering, and hemoglobin abnormalities can also cause inaccurate readings.

Oxyhemoglobin and deoxyhemoglobin are able to absorb infrared and red light at different wavelengths. A pulse oximeter probe emits both infrared and red light via two light-emitting diodes. When the probe is placed across an arterial bed, light is absorbed at the different wavelengths and the percentage of oxygenated hemoglobin with respect to total hemoglobin is expressed – this is denoted SpO_2.

Saturation of 98–100% is normal for SpO_2. The SpO_2 corresponds to a specific number on the hemoglobin–oxygen dissociation curve. The curve slopes down drastically after the SpO_2 drops below 90%. An SpO_2 of 90% corresponds to 60 mmHg on the dissociation curve. At this point, the patient is considered hypoxemic and corrective action needs to be taken.

Temperature Monitoring

Core body temperature should be monitored in all patients under general anesthesia. A simple rectal or a continuously reading rectal thermometer can be used in most patients. Rectal probes are ideal in patients undergoing endoscopic procedures dealing with the respiratory system and nasal and/or oral cavities. Esophageal probes can be utilized when they do not directly interfere with endoscopic procedures. Esophageal probes give a continuous reading and in some cases are combined with an esophageal stethoscope. Core body temperature should be checked and recorded at least every 15 min.

Hypothermia is a by-product of anesthesia but can be prevented with the use of heating pads, forced warm air blankets, and covering the patients with basic items such as fleece pads or bubble wrap. Hypothermia can lead to coagulopathies and increases oxygen consumption due to shivering, with prolonged recovery times and postoperative healing time in general.

Basic Blood Gas Monitoring

Arterial blood gas monitoring is considered the "gold standard" method used to evaluate gas exchange and the acid–base status of the patient. There are many different blood gas analyzers on the market today, ranging from large table-top machines to hand-held bedside machines. Both have their advantages and disadvantages, but the end result is generally the same. Most blood gas analyzers provide, at the minimum, values for pH, $PaCO_2$ (partial pressure of carbon dioxide), PaO_2 (partial pressure of oxygen), SaO_2 (oxygen saturation), and HCO_3^- (bicarbonate level). Other common values include electrolytes, hemoglobin, base excess/deficit, and lactate. An entire chapter could be written on blood gas analysis, hence we will only cover the basics here.

The normal pH in mammals ranges from 7.35 to 7.45. Values below 7.35 indicate acidosis and values above 7.45 indicate alkalosis. As the pH increases, $PaCO_2$ decreases, and as the pH decreases, $PaCO_2$ increases. Therefore, when the $PaCO_2$ levels become elevated (usually from poor ventilation), the pH decreases and the patient develops a respiratory acidosis.

As stated earlier, the normal $ETCO_2$ in mammals is 35–45 mmHg. $ETCO_2$ is an estimate of $PaCO_2$. In mammals, $ETCO_2$ values are generally about 5–7 mmHg lower than the actual $PaCO_2$.

SPECIAL ANESTHETIC CONSIDERATIONS FOR PATIENTS UNDERGOING ENDOSCOPIC PROCEDURES

Rhinoscopy

Rhinoscopic examinations are performed to help diagnose or rule out the presence of fungal or bacterial infections, neoplasia, and the presence of potential foreign bodies. Placing an endoscope into the nasal cavity is very stimulating and biopsies, if taken, can be painful, as shown in Figure 3.5. Full mu-opioids are often used for both premedication and then potentially postoperatively if the procedure is prolonged or painful. Anesthetic induction and monitoring techniques can vary, so drug protocols should be chosen to fit the needs of the individual patient. Infraorbital or maxillary local anesthetic blocks may be helpful in providing a multimodal approach to anesthesia. Local blocks, when performed correctly, block the generation and conduction of nerve impulses. Using local anesthetics is the only way we can provide a complete blockade of pain. Lidocaine and bupivacaine are the two most commonly used local anesthetics. Drug choice should be based on the procedure being performed and the length of time the blockade is desired. Lidocaine has an onset of action of just a few minutes

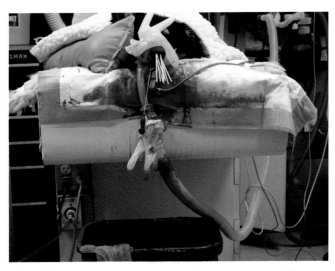

Figure 3.5 Rhinoscopic procedures can cause discomfort and pain. Local blocks can help provide a multimodal approach to anesthesia and may contribute to a smoother recovery.

and a duration of action of about 1–2 h. Bupivacaine has a longer onset of action (10–20 min) and longer duration of action (4–6 h). Postoperative analgesia should be considered at the conclusion of a potentially painful procedure.

Infraorbital Blocks

Infraorbital nerve blocks provide anesthesia to the rostral portion of the maxilla. The opening to the infraorbital canal lies just above the third premolar, as demonstrated in Figure 3.6. After the infraorbital foramen has been palpated, a small needle can then be inserted and advanced into the canal. The needle should advance easily if it is properly placed. If the needle will not advance (likely due to hitting bone), back out slightly, reposition, and start advancing again. Once the needle is properly seated within the canal, aspirate to ensure that the needle is not within a blood vessel. If blood is aspirated, pull out and start again. If nothing is aspirated, it is safe to administer the local anesthetic. Common needle sizes range from 27 to 25 gauge. The length will vary based on the species involved. Cats and brachycephalic dogs have short infraorbital canals, as demonstrated in Figure 3.7. Caution should be exercised with these species because damage to the eye can occur if the needle is advanced too far, as shown in Figure 3.8.

Maxillary blocks

Maxillary nerve blocks provide anesthesia to the upper dental arcade, muzzle, and both the hard and soft palates. This block is best accomplished by inserting

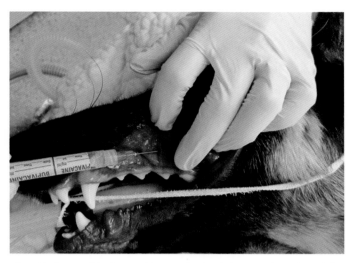

Figure 3.6 Infraorbital nerve blocks provide anesthesia to the rostral portion of the maxilla. The opening to the infraorbital canal lies just above the third premolar and is generally easy to palpate.

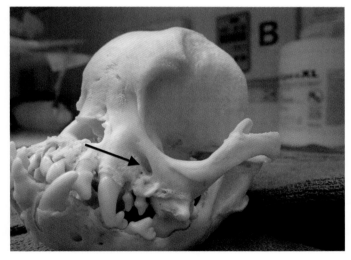

Figure 3.7 Cats and brachycephalic dogs have short infraorbital canals. The arrow points to the opening of the infraorbital canal.

a needle under the rostral portion of the zygomatic arch and directing it in a perpendicular fashion towards the maxillary foramen. Common needle sizes range from 25 to 22 gauge with a length of 1–1.5 in. Table 3.2 lists dose volumes for local anesthetic dental blocks.

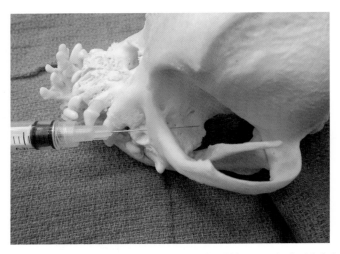

Figure 3.8 The skull of a brachycephalic dog. Caution should be exercised with infraorbital blocks in these species as damage to the eye can occur if the needle is advanced too far. The needle shown is passing through the infraorbital canal.

Table 3.2 Suggested volumes for local anesthetic dental blocks.

Animal	Volume (mL per site)*
Cat and small dog	0.25
Medium-sized dog	0.5
Large to extra-large dog	1.0

*Based on the author's experience. The maximum dose should be calculated prior to administering local anesthetic.
Source: reproduced with permission from Seymour, C. and Duke-Novakovski, T. (eds), *BSAVA Manual of Canine and Feline Anaesthesia and Analgesia*, 2nd edn, 2007. © BSAVA.

Bronchoscopy

Bronchoscopic examinations are commonly performed to help diagnose or rule out the presence of fungal or bacterial infections, neoplasia, asthma, and potential foreign bodies. Owing to the nature of the endoscopic equipment used, anesthesia can become challenging in these patients.

Bronchoscopic procedures are generally not very painful. Butorphanol is often an ideal premedication as it is short acting and usually provides good sedation. Anesthetic induction and monitoring techniques can vary, so drug protocols should be chosen to fit the needs of the individual patient.

Respiratory compromise is often present in these patients, hence oxygen supplementation is important. Most bronchoscopes have a diameter of 5.5 mm and

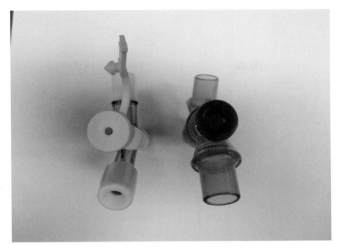

Figure 3.9 Front view of a double-diaphragm adapter, which can be used to provide continuous inhalant anesthesia to the patient and help reduce staff exposure to anesthetic gases. These adapters also allow for proper waste gas scavenging and intermittent positive pressure ventilation (IPPV) if needed.

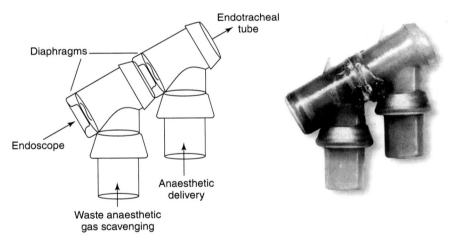

Figure 3.10 Side view of the double-diaphragm adapter in Figure 3.9. Source: reproduced with permission from Seymour, C. and Duke-Novakovski, T. (eds), *BSAVA Manual of Canine and Feline Anaesthesia and Analgesia*, 2nd edn, 2007, Ch. 21, p. 241, diagram 21.6. © BSAVA.

fit through a 7.5 mm or larger endotracheal tube. A double-diaphragm adapter, as shown in Figures 3.9 and 3.10, can be used to provide continuous inhalant anesthesia to the patient and help reduce staff exposure to anesthetic gases. These adapters also allow for proper waste gas scavenging and intermittent positive pressure ventilation (IPPV) if needed.

Anesthetic delivery in smaller patients where the endoscope will not pass through the endotracheal tube or in cases where the double-diaphragm adapter is not available will need to be approached in a different manner.

Most commonly, a large-bore catheter (14 or 16 gauge), small endotracheal tube, or rubber feeding tube is adapted to fit the anesthetic circuit and then placed in the trachea. This will enable to endoscopist to advance the endoscope into the trachea and lower respiratory tract. Oxygen can be delivered using one of these methods, but care must be taken as these small tubes can become kinked or dislodged into the trachea. It is important to note that these methods can contribute to hypercapnia since carbon dioxide is not easily removed and one cannot provide IPPV if the patient becomes apneic during the procedure.

Another oxygen delivery method for smaller patients includes the use of a large-bore catheter attached to a high-frequency jet ventilator, as shown in Figures 3.11 and 3.12. This is the author's preferred method because adequate oxygen supplementation can be administered while providing ventilatory support, thus helping remove the build-up of carbon dioxide. High-frequency jet ventilators provide ultra-low tidal volumes and increased respiratory rates. In the author's experience, most jet ventilators provide appropriate ventilation when the respiratory rate is set to 180 breaths per minute and the pressure is adjusted so that small chest excursions can be noted visually by the anesthetist. $PaCO_2$ levels are generally kept within an acceptable range at these settings.

Regardless of the method chosen for oxygen supplementation, inhalant anesthetics cannot be used due to the lack of a properly sealed airway via the "endotracheal tube." General anesthesia is provided using either intermittent boluses or a constant rate infusion of an anesthetic drug. Propofol is most

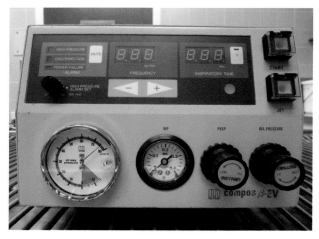

Figure 3.11 High-frequency jet ventilators provide ultra-low tidal volumes and increased respiratory rates.

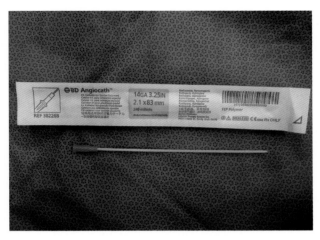

Figure 3.12 Oxygen is delivered to the patient via a large-bore catheter attached to the jet ventilator shown in Figure 3.11.

commonly used and is beneficial because it can be easily titrated to effect, has a rapid onset of action and a short duration of action, and can be delivered as a constant-rate infusion (CRI). In general, canine patients recover well from multiple boluses or CRI administration of propofol. Feline patients, on the other hand, can experience prolonged recoveries after receiving multiple boluses of propofol or CRIs lasting longer than 30 min. Alfaxalone can also be used in a similar manner to a propofol CRI and is often a better option in cats as it has tends to have less negative effects. Box 3.2 provides information for calculating CRIs.

BOX 3.2 CALCULATING A CONSTANT-RATE INFUSION (CRI)

A CRI is a small dose of a drug administered continuously over a period of time. In many instances, CRIs require a loading dose given at the onset of CRI delivery. A loading dose will quickly increase the drug plasma concentration levels, enabling the low-dose CRI to become effective quickly. The induction dose can be used as the loading dose if the CRI is started in the first few minutes after induction.

Calculating a CRI is very easy once you understand what equations to use. For example, let us say you are about to anesthetize a Chihuahua for a bronchoscopic examination with diagnostic sample collection. How would you calculate a CRI of propofol?

The equation for calculating a CRI is as follows:

[(patient′s weight) × (dosage of the drug) × (time factor)]/concentration of the drug

Let the time factor for this equation be 60 min/h.

Let us say the Chihuahua weighs 2.0 kg and the dose of propofol that you are going to start with is 0.2 mg/kg/min (the common dose rage is 0.1–0.4 mg/kg/min). The concentration of propofol is 10 mg/mL.

You now have all the information needed to calculate the CRI using the above equation:

$$[(2.0 \text{ kg}) \times (0.2 \text{ mg/kg/min}) \times (60 \text{ min/h})]/10 \text{ mg/mL} = 2.4 \text{ mL/h}$$

adapted with permission from Seymour, C. and Duke-Novakovski, T. (eds), *BSAVA Manual of Canine and Feline Anaesthesia and Analgesia*, 2nd edn, 2007. © BSAVA.

Monitoring and recovery of the bronchoscopy patient can be difficult. Basic monitoring of vital signs and indirect blood pressure are essential. Placement of an arterial catheter will not only allow for direct blood pressure monitoring, but can also provide information on ventilation and oxygenation status during and after the procedure via blood gas analysis. Pulse oximetry should also be considered as it provides a non-invasive way to help monitor oxygen saturation. Owing to the nature of the procedure, desaturation can occur due to scope placement, fluids in the airway from sample collection, or excessive blood due to biopsy collection. After the procedure has been completed, a normal-sized endotracheal tube should be placed in the trachea and the patient should be provided with oxygen until extubation. Flow-by oxygen support should be provided if necessary during the recovery period. Postoperative pain management should be considered if necessary.

Tracheoscopy

Tracheoscopic procedures are performed to help diagnose or rule out the presence of fungal or bacterial infections, neoplasia, or potential foreign bodies. Depending on the species and size of the patient, a rigid or flexible endoscope may be used. Patients requiring tracheoscopy should be approached in the same manner as the broncoscopic patient.

Esophagoscopy and Gastroduodenoscopy

Esophagoscopy and gastroduodenoscopy are commonly performed in dogs and cats for diagnostic purposes and to facilitate sample collection. Common reasons for esophagoscopy and gastroduodenoscopy include, but are not limited to, foreign body retrieval, biopsy collection, and a minimally invasive way to explore the upper gastrointestinal (GI) tract.

Patients with upper GI disease may present with chronic vomiting, dehydration, poor body condition, electrolyte imbalances, and general malaise. These patients should ideally be rehydrated properly prior to anesthetic induction. Balanced crystalloids are most commonly used for intravenous fluid therapy, but colloids can be administered when necessary. Synthetic colloids are most often given to patients with low proteins, a protein-losing enteropathy or hypovolemia.

Anesthetic protocols will vary based on ASA status, specific procedure performed, drug availability, and clinician preference. Most commonly, patients are given an opioid with or without an anticholinergic. Benzodiazepines or acepromazine can be added to the premedication regime if necessary and appropriate. Patients with a known foreign body should not be given drugs that cause vomiting, hence opioids such as methadone, buprenorphine, or butorphanol are often chosen. A potential negative side effect of opioid administration is an increase in gastroduodenal sphincter tone. An increase in sphincter tone can potentially make it more difficult for the endoscopist to pass the endoscope through the sphincter. In the author's experience, this tends to happen more frequently to lesser experienced persons. Owing to this potential effect, some suggest giving a short-acting, kappa agonist mu antagonist opioid such as butorphanol or not administering any type of opioid until after the procedure has been completed. In the latter situation, the patient can still be provided with analgesia and the opioids may help provide a smoother recovery.

Monitoring parameters are based on the health status of the individual patient. At a minimum, basic monitoring such as heart and respiratory rate, mucus membrane color, capillary refill time, core body temperature, pulse quality, and blood pressure should be performed and recorded every 5 min throughout the procedure. Advanced monitoring techniques such as such direct arterial blood pressure monitoring, central venous pressure, electrocardiography, capnography, pulse oximetry, and so on can be added as needed.

Under most circumstances, these procedures are fairly quick and are not considered very painful. Analgesics are often not needed upon completion of the procedure. In rare cases, removing an esophageal foreign body can cause a pneumomediastinum and pneumothorax. This is often diagnosed by seeing a perforation in the esophagus via the endoscope (or thoracic radiographs). Common signs of a pneumothorax include dyspnea, decreased breath sounds on auscultation, hypoxemia, difficulty providing intermittent positive pressure ventilation, and abnormal expansion of the thoracic cavity. A pulse oximeter can be instrumental in the assessment of oxygenation. If an arterial catheter is in place, a blood gas analysis can be obtained and will give the most accurate account of oxygenation.

Patients who develop a pneumothorax, such as the radiograph shown in Figure 3.13, will likely need thoracocentesis and/or placement of a chest tube(s). In some cases, thoracic surgery may be necessary. Anesthetic management for open thoracic surgery can become difficult. If not already in place, a pulse oximeter, capnograph, and ECG should be set up. An arterial catheter should be placed to obtain continuous blood pressure monitoring and provide easy access to blood gas sampling. Placement of a secondary IV catheter is also ideal as this will provide additional access for bolusing fluids and other drugs. IPPV should be provided once the chest is open. This can be done via manual or mechanical ventilation. Providing IPPV prior to opening the chest can worsen

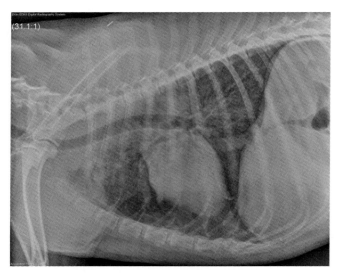

Figure 3.13 This lateral radiograph depicts a classic pneumothorax.

the pneumothorax. Once the chest is opened, negative pressure is lost. Positive end expiratory pressure (PEEP) or continuous positive airway pressure (CPAP) should be applied at this point. PEEP or CPAP applies a chosen constant pressure to the lungs, which keeps the airway from collapsing and helps improve overall oxygenation.

Proper pain management for a patient undergoing thoracic surgery is also important. The thoracoscopy section provides further information regarding analgesia.

Proctoscopy

Proctoscopy is a minimally invasive procedure used to examine the rectum. Proctoscopy enables the clinician to take diagnostic samples and biopsies, and potentially remove foreign bodies without invasive surgery. Under most circumstances, this procedure can usually be performed under heavy sedation. Common premedication combinations include the use of an opioid with or without acepromazine, dexmedetomidine and benzodiazepines.

A dedicated anesthetist should be assigned to the patient even if heavy sedation is planned. The anesthetist should be set up and prepared for general anesthesia in the event that it is necessary. The anesthesia machine, monitoring equipment, and endotracheal tubes should be out and easily within reach. Intravenous catheter placement is suggested. Patients may not require fluid therapy administration, but having IV access is beneficial in the event of an emergency or the need for general anesthesia administration.

Patients under heavy sedation can also benefit from the administration of flow-by oxygen. Basic vital signs such as heart and respiratory rates, pulse quality, core body temperature (if possible), capillary refill time, and observation of mucus membrane color should be taken and recorded at least every 5 min. Recording vital signs, even under heavy sedation, can prove useful as it provides a legal document of the event and it can be accessed if the patient needs to be sedated or anesthetized in the future.

Most proctoscopic procedures are quick and only mildly painful. Postoperative analgesics are generally not necessary.

Colonoscopy

Colonoscopy is a common procedure performed to help facilitate sample collection and diagnose the presence of neoplasia, ulcerations, and generalized lower GI tract disease. There are no special anesthetic considerations for the colonoscopy patient. Anesthesia should be approached in the same manner as with any other case. The overall health status of the patient, including physical examination findings and blood work changes, if any, should be taken into account. An individual plan should be made for each patient. Full mu-opioids are often used as part of the premedication regime. Induction drugs and monitoring equipment are chosen based on the individual needs of the patient. Post-procedural analgesics are often not needed for this procedure, but can be given if necessary.

Vaginoscopy

Vaginoscopy is a minimally invasive procedure used to examine the vagina. Similarly to proctoscopy, vaginoscopy also enables the clinician to take diagnostic samples and biopsies, implant semen, and potentially remove foreign bodies without invasive surgery. With the exception of bitches that present for artificial insemination, the same anesthetic approach as described in the proctoscopy section also applies to vaginoscopy. Bitches in estrous are often not bothered by the vaginoscope and rarely need to be sedated.

Laryngoscopy and Pharyngoscopy

Endoscopy of the larynx and pharynx is performed to help diagnose the presence of neoplasia, bacterial and/or fungal infections, and the presence of a foreign body, assess laryngeal function, and facilitate sample collection. Laryngoscopy can be performed prior to bronchoscopy, rhinoscopy, or esophagogastroduodenoscopic procedures. It is best accomplished just after completion of anesthetic induction but just prior to endotracheal intubation. The larynx is easy to examine and the procedure is usually very quick. Deep, even breaths are needed to assess laryngeal motion adequately. If any abnormality is found, doxapram hydrochloride at a dosage of 0.5–1 mg/kg given intravenously can facilitate deep breathing for a more thorough examination. Flow-by oxygen should be provided when possible and the patient should be immediately intubated upon completion of the examination. The anesthetist should be prepared to administer additional injectable anesthetics in the event that the patient enters a light plane of anesthesia.

Endoscopic examination of the pharynx is also a fairly quick procedure. After induction, the patient is intubated and started on an inhalant anesthetic. Examining the pharynx can be very stimulating to the patient. The anesthetist should be prepared to increase the inhalant or provide additional injectable anesthetics as needed.

When choosing an anesthetic plan, the overall health status of the patient, including physical examination findings and blood work changes, if any, should be taken into account. An individual plan should be made for each patient. Opioids are often used as a part of the premedication regime. Induction drugs and monitoring equipment are chosen based on the individual needs of the patient.

Endoscopic examination of the larynx and pharynx is not general painful. Post-procedural analgesics are not given unless deemed necessary.

Cystoscopy

Cystoscopy is a common procedure performed in dogs and cats to help facilitate sample collection and diagnose the presence of neoplasia, ectopic ureters, and cystic calculi and aid in performing lithotripsy. There are no specific anesthetic considerations for the cystoscopy patient. Anesthesia should be approached in the same manner as with any other case. The overall health status of the patient, including physical examination findings and blood work changes, if any, should be taken into account. An individual plan should be made for each patient. Full mu-opioids are often used as part of the premedication regime with or without an anticholinergic. Induction drugs and monitoring equipment are chosen based on the individual needs of the patient. Post-procedural analgesics are given if needed and are based on the procedural time frame and potential pain caused.

Thoracoscopic and laparoscopic procedures

Laparoscopic and thoracoscopic procedures utilizing rigid endoscopy have become more commonplace in veterinary medicine over the last several years. Minimally invasive techniques provide a way for the surgeon not only to obtain internal organ biopsies, but also to perform major surgical procedures that were previously possible only by traditional surgical intervention. Patients tend to have a much quicker recovery and often experience less pain when minimally invasive techniques are used.

Thoracoscopy

Thoracoscopy is utilized for obtaining diagnostic samples such as tissue biopsies and for a minimally invasive surgical approach and intervention. Common thoracoscopic surgeries include, but are not limited to, lung lobectomy, pericardiectomy, mass removal, and repair of vascular ring anomalies.

Thoracoscopic procedures are performed by first placing access ports in the thoracic cavity. Ports allow the surgeons to pass a rigid endoscope, instruments, and insufflate gas such as air or CO_2. The introduction of gas causes a pneumothorax and allows for better visualization of the intrathoracic structures.

Anesthetic considerations are similar to those in patients requiring an open lateral thoracotomy or median sternotomy. The use of IPPV and PEEP is essential once the thoracic cavity has been penetrated and negative pressure is lost. PEEP reduces atelectasis and hypoxemia by keeping the lung slightly and continuously inflated throughout the procedure. PEEP is most often provided via a valve (shown in Figure 3.14) that can be added to any anesthesia machine. In some cases, PEEP is a standard mode that can be dialed in on a mechanical ventilator. Advanced monitoring equipment should be used throughout the procedure including, but not limited to, SpO_2, $ETCO_2$, ECG, arterial blood gas sampling, and direct arterial blood pressure.

Although thoracoscopy is considered a minimally invasive procedure, discomfort is still caused by the port placement and the surgery itself. Insufflating the thoracic cavity is also uncomfortable. Full mu-opioids are suggested as a premedication with or without the addition of an anticholinergic. Anesthetic induction can vary, so drug protocols should be chosen to fit the needs of the individual patient. Balanced or multimodal anesthetic techniques such as an analgesic CRI can be utilized during thoracoscopic procedures. Common drugs used for an analgesic CRI generally include morphine or fentanyl with or without the addition of ketamine and/or lidocaine. The addition of a CRI not only provides analgesia, but can also reduce the overall inhalant anesthetic requirements.

One-lung ventilation

Thoracoscopic procedures often require the use of selective one-lung ventilation. As its name suggests, one-lung ventilation allows for only one lung to be ventilated at a given time. This is advantageous for the surgeon because it allows the lung requiring surgery to remain collapsed during the procedure. One-lung ventilation can also provide better visualization for the surgeons during an intrathoracic procedure. Desaturation and hypoxemia can occur during one-lung ventilation. As with any open thoracic procedure, advanced monitoring techniques should be used and include, but are not limited to, $ETCO_2$, SpO_2, ECG, direct arterial blood pressure monitoring, and arterial blood gas sampling.

Two main methods are used to achieve one-lung ventilation. The first includes the use of a double-lumen Robertshaw endobronchial tube, shown in Figures 3.15a and b. This specialized tube is comprised of a long and a short tube with two separate cuffs. The tubes come in left- and right-sided versions. Owing to the lung anatomy of the dog, the left-sided tube is generally used. The long portion of the tube is inserted into the left mainstem bronchus. After

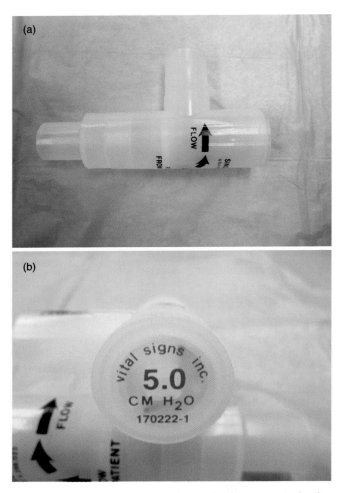

Figure 3.14 The use of IPPV and PEEP is essential once the thoracic cavity has been penetrated and negative pressure is lost. PEEP reduces atelectasis and hypoxemia by keeping the lung slightly and continuously inflated throughout the procedure. PEEP is most often provided via a valve as shown here that can be added to any anesthesia machine.

both cuffs are inflated properly, the left and right lungs are functionally isolated from each other, as shown in Figure 3.15c. Blind placement of the tube is often not successful; therefore, the use of an bronchoscope is suggested. The bronchoscope should be passed through both lumens of the tube to ensure proper placement within the trachea. Robertshaw tubes are manufactured for human use, hence they tend to be short and do not work very well in canine patients over 20–25 kg.

The second method commonly used for one-lung ventilation is via an endobronchial blocker, shown in Figure 3.15d. A special three-port adapter is attached

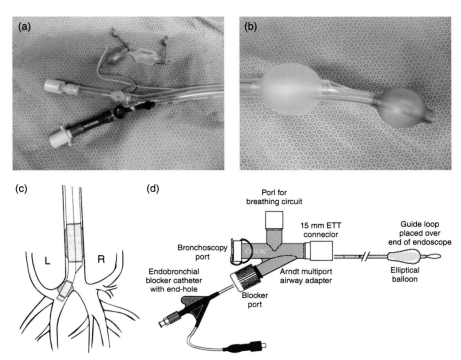

Figure 3.15 One-lung ventilation can be accomplished using a double-lumen Robertshaw endobronchial tube. The Robertshaw tube is comprised of a long and a short tube with two separate cuffs. The long portion of the tube is generally inserted into the left mainstem bronchus. After both cuffs are inflated properly, the left and right lungs are functionally isolated from each other. Source: parts (c) and (d) reproduced with permission from Seymour, C. and Duke-Novakovski, T. (eds), *BSAVA Manual of Canine and Feline Anaesthesia and Analgesia*, 2nd edn, 2007, Ch. 21, pp. 230 and 240, respectively. © BSAVA.

to a standard endotracheal tube. The circuit attaches to one side of the adapter and allows for normal inhalant delivery. The bronchoscope is passed through the middle portion of the adapter and allows for visualization and proper placement of the endobronchial blocker. The endobronchial blocker is passed through the second side port. The endobronchial blocker is looped onto the end of the bronchoscope and passed into the trachea. Once the endobronchial blocker is properly seated within the bronchus, it can be inflated and the bronchoscope removed.

Laparoscopy

Laparoscopy is often used to collect diagnostic samples such as tissue biopsies and perform major surgical procedures including, but not limited to, adrenalectomy, splenectomy, abdominal mass removal, cholecystectomy, and laparoscopic-assisted ovariectomy. As discussed in the thoracoscopy section, procedures are performed by first placing access ports into the abdominal cavity. Ports allow the surgeons to pass a rigid endoscope and instruments, and insufflate gas such as air or CO_2. The introduction of gas causes the abdomen to expand, allowing for better visualization of internal organs and vascular structures. Insufflation of gas into the abdomen increases intra-abdominal pressure, thus placing pressure on the diaphragm and making it difficult for the patient to breathe effectively. IPPV is required during this portion of the procedure.

Anesthetic considerations are similar to those in patients requiring an open celiotomy. Although laparoscopy is considered a minimally invasive procedure, discomfort is still caused by the port placement and the surgery itself. Insufflating the abdomen is also uncomfortable. Full mu-opioids are generally used as a premedication with or without the addition of an anticholinergic. Anesthetic induction and monitoring techniques can vary, so drug protocols should be chosen to fit the needs of the individual patient. Balanced or multimodal anesthetic techniques such as an epidural and/or an analgesic CRI can be utilized during laparoscopic procedures as needed. Common drugs used for epidural analgesia include either a local anesthetic, an opioid such as preservative-free morphine, or a combination of the two. Common drugs used for an analgesic CRI generally include morphine or fentanyl with or without the addition of ketamine and/or lidocaine. The addition of a CRI not only provides analgesia, but can also reduce the overall inhalant anesthetic requirements. Since laparoscopy is a minimally invasive procedure, the use of an epidural if often unnecessary in most cases.

Arthroscopy

Arthroscopic procedures are commonly used to help diagnose the presence of and treat disease within the joint. Although arthroscopy is minimally invasive, the procedure itself is still considered to be somewhat painful. Patients are generally premedicated utilizing full mu-opioids with or without an anticholinergic. Anesthetic induction and monitoring techniques can vary, so drug protocols should be chosen to fit the needs of the individual patient. A multimodal approach to anesthesia is suggested for arthroscopic procedures. Locoregional techniques such as epidural analgesia/anesthesia and local blockades can provide both pain relief and MAC reduction throughout the procedure and in some cases provide postoperative analgesia. Postoperative pain relief is generally administered at the conclusion of the procedure. In most cases, full mu-opioids are suggested.

Epidural placement is relatively easy to perform and takes only a few minutes when administered by an experienced anesthetist. The patient is generally placed in sternal recumbency, as shown in Figure 3.16, although lateral recumbency is also an option. The spine should be straight and symmetric with the hind legs pulled forward and positioned against the sides of the abdomen. Pulling the legs forward will help open the epidural space. The wings of the ilium should first be

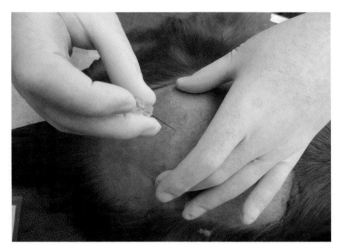

Figure 3.16 The epidural space is located between vertebral bodies L7 and S1. The wings of the ilium can be palpated and used as landmarks to help identify the epidural space.

palpated. The lumbosacral space can be palpated between vertebral bodies L7 and S1. Prior to placing the epidural needle, the area should be shaved and aseptically prepared. Sterile gloves must be worn when administering the epidural. A 25- or 22-gauge spinal needle is generally suggested. The spinal needle is placed on the midline, perpendicular to the skin, and slowly inserted into the epidural space. A "pop" is often felt as the needle passes through the ligamentum flavum and enters the epidural space. If the needle hits bone, you have gone too far and need to back the needle out slightly. A sterile glass syringe containing a small amount of air should be placed on the spinal needle and injected into the space. If air injects easily then you are in the correct spot. If there is a vacuum on the syringe you are not in the correct space and need to reposition the needle. You can also use a technique called the hanging drop technique. Once you have placed the spinal needle through the skin, you can place a drop of saline into the hub of the needle. Slowly advance the needle into the epidural space. The drop of saline will be sucked into the hub of the spinal needle once you are in the correct space. If the drop of saline is not sucked into the spinal needle, you are likely not in the epidural space. Once the needle is correctly placed, you can attach the syringe with the drugs in it onto the spinal needle. Always aspirate back to ensure there is no blood or spinal fluid present. If blood is aspirated you need to pull out and start over. If spinal fluid is aspirated, you should only deliver about one-quarter of the initial calculated dose. Common drugs used for epidural administration include preservative-free morphine, lidocaine, bupivacaine, and buprenorphine. Local anesthetics and opioids can also be used in combination with each other. Epidural anesthesia/analgesia should not be administered if the patient is septic or has signs of pyoderma or a skin infection around the epidural site.

POSTOPERATIVE MANAGEMENT

Postoperative analgesia should be provided when a painful procedure has been performed. Common postoperative drugs include full mu-opioids, partial agonists such as buprenorphine, kappa agonist mu antagonist opioids such as butorphanol, and non-steroidal anti-inflammatory drugs (NSAIDs). NSAIDs used in conjunction with opioid administration help provide multimodal analgesia and should only be used in healthy patients (those with no evidence of kidney or liver disease) not concurrently receiving steroids.

Ideally, the postoperative patient should recover in a warm, low-stress environment. After extubation, the heart rate, respiratory rate, core body temperature, and pain should be assessed by a dedicated veterinary technician at least every 30 min. Patients should be monitored until they are fully recovered and able to maintain body temperature without heat support. It is suggested that more critical patients have continuous monitoring for several hours to a few days postoperatively.

Table 3.3 contains a list of common drugs with dosages to help formulate a balanced anesthetic plan for every phase of the procedure. Utilizing this table along with the anesthesia techniques outlined in this chapter will make the procedure easier, and result in a smoother, uneventful recovery for the patient.

Table 3.3   Common dosages of pre- and post-anesthetic drugs.

Class	Drugs*
Full mu-opioids	Hydromorphone 0.05–1.0 mg/kg SC, IM, IV Morphine 0.3–1.0 mg/kg SC, IM, IV Methadone 0.2–0.5 mg/kg SC, IM, IV Oxymorphone 0.02–0.06 mg/kg SC, IM, IV
Partial agonists	Buprenorphine 10–20 µg/kg IM, IV
Mixed agonists	Butorphanol 0.2–0.4 mg/kg SC, IM, IV
Anticholinergics	Atropine 0.02–0.04 mg/kg SC, IM Glycopyrrolate 0.01–0.02 mg/kg SC, IM
α_2-Agonists	Dexmedetomidine 5–7.5 µg/kg (cat) and 2.5–5 µg/kg IM (dog)
α_2-Antagonists	Atipamezole: 10 times the dose of dexmedetomidine (administer same volume as dexmedetomidine) IM
Phenothiazines	Acepromazine 0.01–0.05 mg/kg
Dissociatives	Ketamine 5–10 mg/kg SC, IM Telazol 2–3 mg/kg SC, IM (cat) and 4–5 mg/kg SC, IM (dog)
Common induction agents	Propofol 6–8 mg/kg IV Propofol 4 mg/kg + midazolam 0.3 mg/kg IV Propofol 4 mg/kg + diazepam 0.3 mg/kg IV Propofol 4 mg/kg + ketamine 2 mg/kg IV

Table 3.3 (*Continued*).

Class	Drugs*
	Alfaxalone 1-2 mg/kg + midazolam 0.1 to 0.3 mg/kg Ketamine 5 mg/kg + midazolam 0.3 mg/kg Ketamine 5 mg/kg + diazepam 0.5 mg/kg Fentanyl 10 µg/kg + midazolam 0.3 mg/kg Fentanyl 10 µg/kg + diazepam 0.5 mg/kg Etomidate 1.5 mg/kg + midazolam 0.3 mg/kg Etomidate 1.5 mg/kg + diazepam 0.5 mg/kg
Constant-rate infusions:	
Cats: fentanyl loading dose 5 µg/kg	CRI 0.2–0.4 µg/kg/min
Dogs: fentanyl loading dose 5–10 µg/kg/min	CRI 0.5–0.7 µg/kg/min
Propofol	CRI 0.2–0.4 mg/kg/min
Alfaxalone 0.1-0.3 mg/kg/min	

*Drug protocols should be tailored to each individual patient. Debilitated, pediatric, and geriatric patients may require smaller doses than those animals that are considered healthy. These are the drug doses commonly used at the UC Davis Veterinary Medical Teaching Hospital.

SUGGESTED READING

Bryant, S. (ed.) (2010) *Anesthesia for Veterinary Technicians*. Blackwell Publishing, Ames, IA.

Seymour, C. and Duke-Novakovski, T. (eds) (2007) *BSAVA Manual of Canine and Feline Anaesthesia and Analgesia*, 2nd edn. British Small Animal Veterinary Association, Gloucester.

Tranquilli, W.J., Thurmon, J.C., and Grimm, K.A. (eds) (2007) *Lumb & Jones' Veterinary Anesthesia and Analgesia*, 4th edn. Blackwell Publishing, Ames, IA.

4 Upper gastrointestinal tract endoscopy

Susan Cox

William R. Pritchard Veterinary Medical Teaching Hospital, University of California-Davis, Davis,California, USA

The endoscopic examination of the gastrointestinal (GI) tract includes the esophagus, stomach and duodenum. Upper GI tract examinations include all three areas, termed esophagogastroduodenoscopy (EGD). EGD and lower GI endoscopy can be performed consecutively, depending on clinical signs.

The technician plays a pivotal role in upper GI endoscopy, particularly in biopsy sampling, documentation and foreign body retrieval. Usually that same technician is monitoring the patient under anesthesia, so performing both tasks can be challenging. Understanding the fundamentals of GI endoscopy will enable the technician to anticipate what the endoscopist will require, which allows more time to concentrate on the patient during the procedure.

Specialized equipment and technical assistance are needed for upper GI studies such as esophageal stricture procedures, foreign body retrievals and percutaneous endoscopic gastrostomy (PEG) tube placements. These procedures are discussed in depth in this chapter.

PATIENT PREPARATION

For optimal visualization in upper gastrointestinal (UGI) procedures in the canine or feline, food should be withheld from the patient 12–24 h before the procedure, or longer if delayed gastric emptying is suspected. If a bleeding disorder is suspected, a coagulation panel (PT/PTT, fibrinogen) should be included with the minimum database. Barium sulfate used for UGI studies can plug endoscope channels; it is advisable to delay an EGD by 12–24 h and take a radiograph demonstrating no barium in the patient's GI tract. If an emergency situation demands GI endoscopy, endoscope suction should be avoided and immediate post-procedure endoscope processing should be implemented.

Locating the antrum may be difficult in patients that have had a gastropexy procedure. It may be beneficial to place the patient in right lateral recumbency and insufflate for improved visualization.

EQUIPMENT AND INSTRUMENTATION

Flexible endoscopes are used for EGD procedures. Although some gastroscopes have two-way deflection, four-way deflection provides easier maneuverability in the stomach. All gastroscopes should have functioning air/water and suction capabilities. For size recommendations, see Table 4.1. Gastroscopes with the correct proportions provide the endoscopist with a manageable outer diameter for pyloral intubations, and also the ability to obtain sizable diagnostic biopsy samples. Sigmoidoscopes, or rigid proctoscopes, can be used for extraction of esophageal foreign bodies, such as fishhooks.

Flexible forceps are used for biopsy and foreign body retrieval. Spiked forceps are not generally used in GI endoscopy as they crush cells, yielding poor diagnostic samples, although they may be useful in obtaining biopsies of tough esophageal tissue. Forceps for retrieval of foreign bodies are varied in their design, depending on what is to be retrieved, and their application will be discussed later in this chapter. Guarded cytology brushes and aspiration tubing to collect duodenal fluid may also be used for sample collection.

Esophageal strictures require the use of sets of balloon dilators with guidewires. Esophageal dilator sizes start at 6 mm and progress to 20 mm. A balloon inflation system can provide accurate pressure measurements at the stricture site.

PEG tube kits are commercially available in sizes 18 and 24 French gauge (Fr) inner diameter and are complete with the PEG tube, bumper, IV catheter-type introducer and feeding adapter. PEG tubes can also be purchased singly and adapted for endoscopic use with a loop of suture coming out of a tapered end. Two types of PEG tubes are shown in Figure 4.1. For a list of supplies needed, see Box 4.1.

Table 4.1   Patient size versus endoscope size for upper gastrointestinal endoscopy procedures

Species/weight	Outer diameter (mm)	Working length (m)	Channel size (mm)*
Feline	7.9	1.4	2.0
Canine <10 kg	7.9	1.4	2.0
Canine 10–20 kg	8.5	2.0	2.8
Canine >20 kg	10.0	2.1	2.8

*Instruments should be 0.2 mm smaller than channel size. For example, a 2 mm channel will accept a 1.8 mm instrument.

BOX 4.1 SUPPLIES NEEDED FOR PEG TUBES

- Flexible endoscope
- Air/water cleaning adapter
- Water bottle
- Suction unit
- Component tower
  - Monitor on
  - Camera or processor and light source
    - Patient info. entered
    - Insufflation/air buttons depressed
    - Ignition button depressed
      - White balance performed
    - Water bottle/suction attached
  - Image capture
    - Patient info. entered
- Non-bacteriostatic lube
- Mouth speculae
- Warm water bowl for pre- and post-scope check
- Examination gloves and gown
- Biopsy forceps
- Foreign body
  - Retrieval forceps
- 4 × 4 gauze sponges with saline
- Esophageal stricture
  - Balloon dilators/bougies
  - Guidewires
  - Corticosteroid injection
  - Balloon inflation system with saline
- PEG tube placement
  - PEG tube kit
  - Suture
  - Stockinette
  - Sterile gloves
  - Clippers and surgical scrub
  - Cable ties
  - Feeding adapter
- Biopsy supplies
  - Biopsy cassettes
  - Formalin jars/culture media
  - Needle for biopsy transfer to cassettes
  - Paperwork for biopsy processing
- Endoscopy report to record observations during procedure

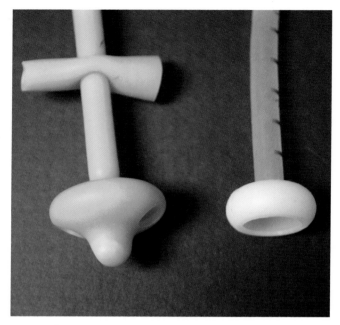

Figure 4.1 Two types of PEG tubes are shown. The tube on the left is a latex Pezzer mushroom-tipped catheter. These catheters are cheaper than silicone, but need to be adapted to use with an endoscope. The tube on the right is a silicone button open-end catheter. These tubes come in a pre-made kit in either 20 or 24 Fr sizes.

PROCEDURE

- General anesthesia
- Left lateral recumbency
  ○ Places antrum/pylorus dorsal for easier examination and entry, as shown in Figure 4.2
- Mouth speculum on right canine teeth (see Figures 4.2 and 4.3)
  ○ Cut-off syringe barrel may be more beneficial in felines (see Suggested reading)
- Oropharyngeal examination
  ○ Check tonsils-in/out of tonsilar fossae
  ○ Palpate hard/soft palate, check under tongue – masses, foreign material
  ○ Brief dental examination
- Endoscope
  ○ Test suction, air/water capabilities, image on monitor
- Esophagus
  ○ Upper esophageal sphincter dorsal to endotracheal tube
  ○ Technician may need to digitally occlude the esophagus caudal to the larynx for adequate insufflation and subsequent visualization

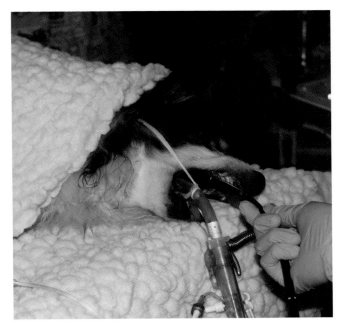

Figure 4.2 Patient positioning for an EGD procedure. The patient is placed in left lateral recumbency, and a mouth speculum is placed on the left canine teeth. The endoscope is placed dorsal to the endotracheal tube, with the neck slightly extended.

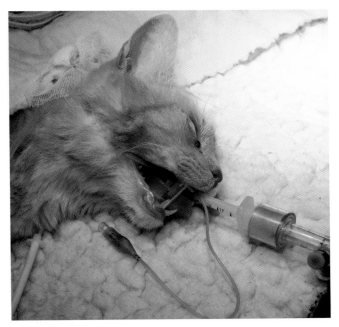

Figure 4.3 A 1 mL syringe barrel is used as a mouth speculum in a feline patient. These can be made to any length. Soft tubing may also be placed on the ends.

- ○ Lower esophageal sphincter (LES) – located at the gastro–esophageal junction
- ○ Standard appearance
  - ▪ Mucosa pale pink, minimal to no fluid present
  - ▪ Felines – distinctive ring pattern on inner wall diameter (see Figure 4.4)
- ○ Abnormal Findings
  - ▪ Neoplasia – leiomyomas at LES, sarcomas, carcinomas (see Figure 4.5)
  - ▪ Strictures
    - – See Stricture treatment later in the chapter
  - ▪ Foreign bodies (see Figure 4.6)
  - ▪ Inflammation
- ○ Challenging to biopsy
- Stomach
  - ○ 5 areas (starting proximally) – cardia, fundus, body (includes the greater curvature), angulus, antrum (includes pylorus)
  - ○ Minimal endoscopic insufflation
    - ▪ Easier to intubate pylorus
    - ▪ Stable anesthetized patient (see Chapter 3)
  - ○ Standard appearance
    - ▪ Mucosa – smooth, pink, glistening
    - ▪ Rugal folds (see Figure 4.13)
      - – Mucosa at greater curvature
      - – Disappear with insufflation
      - – Prime site for biopsies

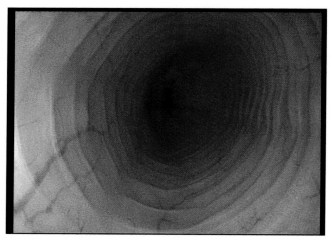

Figure 4.4 Grossly normal esophagus in a feline patient. A distinctive herringbone pattern is evident within the pale pink mucosa. The lower esophageal sphincter is seen distally.

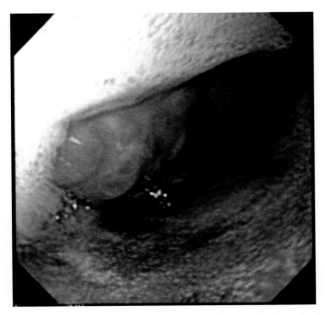

Figure 4.5 The esophagus of a Chow Chow, looking towards the LES. Note the dark pigmentation on the esophageal mucosa, which is normal for this breed. This patient also has multiple masses on the left side of the image.

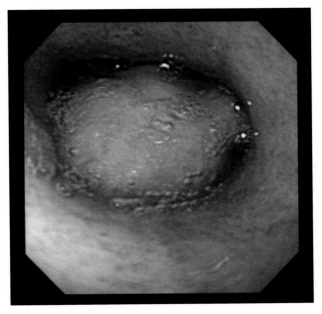

Figure 4.6 An apple core wedged in the esophagus of a canine. Esophageal foreign bodies can be difficult to remove, depending on the time of ingestion and the shape of the object. Esophageal perforation can occur and require surgical correction.

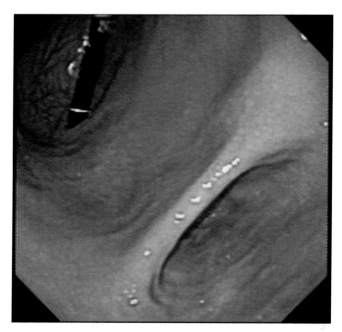

Figure 4.7 A retroflex view in the stomach. The endoscope is flexed around the greater curvature so that the cardia, incisura and antrum can be observed. When performing a biopsy, biopsy forceps should be placed in the instrument channel before the retroflex maneuver is performed.

- ▪ J-maneuver, or endoscope retroflexion (see Figure 4.7)
  - – Allows visualization of fundus and cardia
  - – For biopsy, forceps in endoscope prior to retroflexion
    - ▫ Less force placed on biopsy channel
- ○ Fasted patient
  - ▪ Small amount of liquid expected
  - ▪ Minimal amount of Food or bile present
    - – Bilious fluid indicates Reflux from pylorus
- ○ Pyloric sphincter
  - ▪ Normally closed, but not significant if gaping slightly
  - ▪ Smaller biopsies obtained compared with other areas of stomach due to a ring of tough smooth muscle
  - ▪ Endoscopic pyloral intubation
    - – If intubation is difficult, the technician can pass biopsy forceps through pylorus to act as guidewire for endoscope to slide over (forceps in closed position)

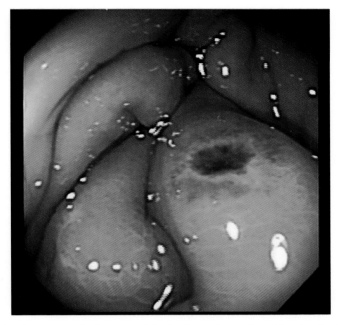

Figure 4.8 An ulcer present in the stomach body of a canine patient. Biopsies should be taken at the edge to avoid the necrotic center.

- Remove endoscope, place patient in sternal or right lateral recumbency
- If unsuccessful, blind biopsies performed
  - □ Flexible forceps passed through pylorus
- ○ Abnormal findings
  - ▪ Foreign objects
  - ▪ bile
    - Reflux from pylorus
  - ▪ Ulcers – erosive/hyperemic mucosa (see Figure 4.8)
  - ▪ Polyps
  - ▪ Masses (see Figure 4.9)
- ○ Biopsy sites
  - ▪ Note tissue friability
  - ▪ Note abnormal bleeding from sites post biopsy
- • Duodenum
  - ○ Standard appearance
    - ▪ Slightly paler and more granular than stomach mucosa
    - ▪ Major and minor duodenal papilla (see Figure 4.10)
      - Approximately 5 cm from pyloral entrance

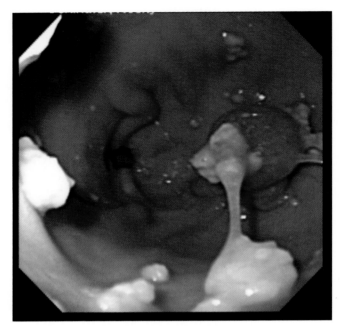

Figure 4.9 The antrum is an area of the stomach that contains the pyloric sphincter, which leads to the duodenum. Biopsy samples tend to be smaller around the pylorus due to tough musculature. A polypoid mass is also present on the right of the image.

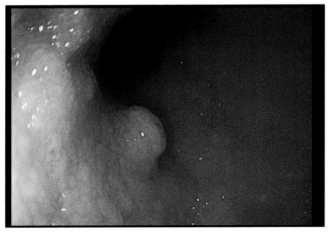

Figure 4.10 The major duodenal papilla, seen in the middle of the image, is located approximately 5 cm from the pylorus. The minor duodenal papilla is also located here. Biopsies of this area should be avoided.

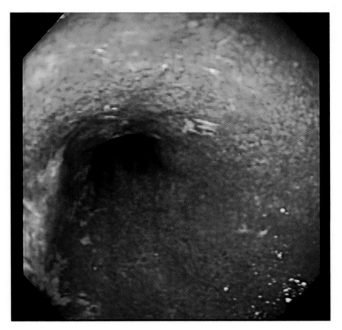

Figure 4.11 Abnormal duodenal mucosa in a canine patient. Note the increased granularity and hyperemia of the mucosal wall.

- - Can appear slightly raised on mucosal surface
  - - Avoid biopsying
  - ■ Peyer's patches – round areas of lymphoid tissue along mucosa
- ○ Abnormal Findings (see Figure 4.11)
  - ■ Enteritis and IBD diagnosed histologically based on degree of severity
  - ■ Mucosal changes
    - - Granularity
    - - Friability
      - □ Excessive bleeding with endoscope contact
      - □ Abnormal bleeding post biopsy
  - ■ Neoplasia may appear obstructive
  - ■ Lymphangectasia
    - - Appearance
      - □ Milky white mucosal surface
      - □ Sloughs easily with endoscope contact
    - - Severity of disease diagnosed via histopathology
- • Biopsies taken retrograde (see Sample collection and processing)
- • Air removed from stomach and esophagus after biopsies performed.
- • Encourage endoscopist to complete endoscopy report

ESOPHAGEAL STRICTURE TREATMENT UTILIZING ENDOSCOPY

Stricture treatment can be performed using endoscopy to diagnose, assess severity of the stricture, and guide the placement of dilation catheter balloons. Clients should be informed that stricture dilation procedures should be performed every 2–4 days or until clinical signs (regurgitation, etc.) have abated and the stricture is significantly reduced.

The technician plays a key role in treating strictures – keeping accurate records on stricture location, length, dilator/guidewire sizes used, placing the dilator within the stricture, and dilation times will aid in treatment and result in shorter anesthesia times for the subsequent procedures. The technician must also watch for gastric overdistension with insufflation. Technical staff can also discuss nutritional needs and medical at-home management with clients.

Procedure

- General anesthesia
- Left lateral recumbency
- Mouth speculum on right canine teeth
- Stricture(s) identified
  - Measurements
    - Stricture location
      - From tip of nose to stricture
    - Total stricture length
      - Post-dilation with endoscope
  - Intralesional corticosteroid injections
    - Endoscopic injection needle through the biopsy channel
      - Pre-load drug into needle; use saline to inject
    - Injected at four sites circumferentially
    - Dose: 0.4 mg/kg or 0.5–1.0 mL divided
  - Balloon dilation
    - Well-lubricated dilator placed at stricture site
      - Option – guidewire placed alongside endoscope and visualized at stricture site, then the dilator is passed over the guidewire
    - Middle of dilator balloon at midpoint of stricture, as shown in Figure 4.12
    - Inflated to recommended pressure points with inflation device; refer to balloon packaging instructions or endoscopist's preference
    - Radial pressure maintained for 1–3 min intervals
      - Increased radial pressure and/or larger balloon dilators may be needed as stricture is dilated

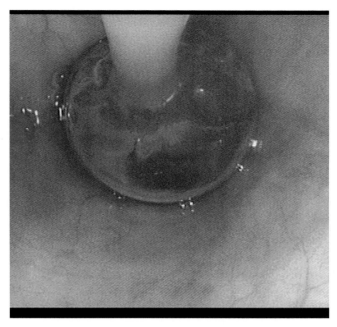

Figure 4.12 Balloon dilation of an esophageal stricture. Saline is used to inflate the balloon to achieve radial pressure at the site. The esophagus is carefully monitored for perforation after each session. A small amount of bloody discharge may be seen at the site.

- Observations
  - Excessive bleeding
  - Tearing of friable mucosa
  - Esophageal perforation
- Record for future procedures
  - Balloon size(s)
  - Pressure measurements
  - Time increments
- Remove air and excessive fluid from stomach and esophagus

ENDOSCOPIC FOREIGN BODY RETRIEVAL

Many foreign bodies in the esophagus and stomach may be safely removed with endoscopy. A faster recovery time and a less invasive approach make endoscopy the procedure of choice over surgical intervention for most foreign bodies encountered.

Foreign bodies initially observed on radiographs more than 8 h old should be radiographed again. Some foreign bodies will travel into the duodenum and require surgery or monitoring and may pass through the gastrointestinal tract without complication. Foreign bodies such as bones, fishhooks, or rawhide chews that are lodged in the esophagus are painful and should be retrieved as soon as possible. Toxic objects such as coins (pennies minted after 1982 cause zinc toxicity) and other metal objects should also be swiftly removed. Smooth or large round objects such as corncobs and heavy items are difficult to get through the LES and should not be attempted. Excessive food in the stomach makes visualization and retrieval of foreign bodies difficult. If possible, the procedure should be delayed.

Communication with owners regarding post-procedure complications is vital. Patients after esophageal foreign body removal should be monitored for signs of esophageal strictures, such as difficulty/painful swallowing and regurgitation. These patients may also require nutritional management and, in some cases, a gastrostomy tube may need to be placed until the site heals. If endoscopic retrieval is unsuccessful, surgical intervention may be necessary, which may require additional anesthesia time with increased expense.

Instrumentation is varied for the type of foreign body to be retrieved. The actual foreign body removal procedure may take little time, especially if the object is radiographically identified and the correct instrumentation is available and in working order. The endoscopist and technician should approach this procedure as a team – knowing exactly when to open and/or close an instrument around a foreign object can turn a long and difficult procedure into a short and successful one.

Patient preparation is the same as for an EGD. The esophageal foreign body could prevent air from escaping through the oral cavity, so watch for gastric distension. When the foreign body is discovered in the esophagus, the surrounding mucosa should first be assessed, and insufflation should be carefully monitored. Damaged mucosa around the object could tear if handled aggressively or pressure becomes excessive.

It is often difficult to maneuver retrieval forceps within the esophagus. It may help to push the foreign body *carefully* into the stomach in order to grasp it more securely, or let gastric juices in the stomach digest the object (bones, rawhide chews, etc.).

Knowing which forceps to use on various objects comes with experience. Knowing how and where to grasp a foreign body to get it through the LES is also a skill that is mastered in time, and requires good communication between endoscopist and technician. Once the object is securely grasped, the forceps should be retracted with the foreign body moved as close to the endoscope as possible, with the technician holding the forceps closed with one hand and keeping tension on the forceps at the biopsy channel port with the other hand. This maneuver allows the endoscope/foreign body to be removed as one unit, making it easier to pass through the LES and upper esophageal sphincter (UES).

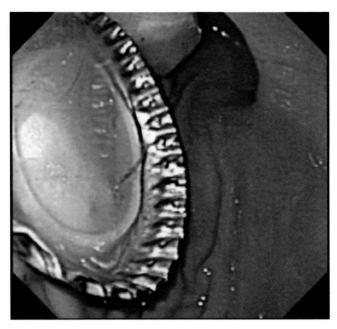

Figure 4.13 A metal bottle cap and rock in the stomach body of a canine patient. The bottle cap was easily removed with rat-tooth retrieval forceps (see Chapter 1) – the crimped edges provide a firm hold. A single-loop snare was used to extract the rock.

Flexible retrieval forceps to be kept on hand include an oval loop snare, rat tooth, and three- or four-pronged graspers. Most of these forceps are designed to be single-use, so purchasing at least two of each kind can be beneficial. Objects with a crimped or raised edge or ridge (see Figure 4.13) are the easiest to remove – the edge is easily gripped by rat-tooth or pronged grasping forceps (see Chapter 1). Try to snare sharp-edged objects so that the edges are behind the grasped portion. If the object was snared with single-loop forceps and is dropped in the esophagus, a pronged grasper may be required to bring it into the oral cavity, so having a variety of retrieval forceps is essential. Fishhooks should be removed carefully. A large-diameter proctoscope with long laparoscopic forceps can shield the fishhook from the esophageal mucosa once the fishhook is freed. Circular objects with a hole in the middle may be removed by passing a long strand of umbilical tape or nylon suture through the hole using retrieval forceps, regrasping the string on the other side, and carefully bringing it up and out of the oral cavity. The endoscope can be used as a visual aid if necessary.

Radiographs are not always reliable, especially if multiple foreign objects are suspected or the object is radiopaque, so be sure to review all areas in the stomach for any hidden objects. Remove all air from the stomach before withdrawing the endoscope. Be sure to document any abnormal findings. Biopsies may also be indicated of any suspicious areas.

For further details regarding retrieval procedures, consult the Suggested reading list.

PEG TUBE PLACEMENT

Percutaneous endoscopic gastrostomy (PEG) tubes are used in those patients with normal GI motility that cannot meet caloric requirements. PEG tubes are placed in animals under general anesthesia, so it may be necessary initially to place a nasogastric tube to stabilize the debilitated patient. PEG tube placements require two individuals – an endoscopist and a technician to assist with placement location and tube handling.

Discussion with clients regarding PEG tube care is critical. Patients with PEG tubes require a major time commitment – blending food, tube feedings, and tube care are performed two or three times per day. A PEG tube that is inadvertently removed is considered an emergency situation and the patient should be seen immediately. Client handouts are helpful and should outline how to feed through the PEG tube, and also how much to feed and possible complications.

It is not recommended to place a PEG tube endoscopically in a dog larger than 20 kg, as the weight of the stomach causes the stomach mucosa to fall off the PEG tube (PEG tubes in these patients may be surgically placed). If not discovered, peritonitis could occur from accidental food administration. After an 8–12 week duration and a stoma has formed between the skin and the stomach wall, PEG tubes can be replaced with a low-profile gastrostomy device (LPGD).

Procedure

- General anesthesia
- Right lateral recumbency
  - Places antrum dorsally
- Clip and surgical scrub – left side
  - Last two ribs including left flank
- Endoscope passed into stomach
  - Visualize antrum
  - Insufflate to displace organs between stomach and body wall
- Choose site for PEG stoma
  - Technician applies digital pressure beside last rib with sterile gloved hands
  - Optimum site antrum/body wall junction
  - Prethread needle/catheter – 1-0 suture material
- 18 Fr needle or IV catheter inserted through stomach wall and push suture through until 3–4 cm visible
  - Retract endoscope slightly prior to insertion

- Grab suture end with biopsy forceps, pull endoscope/forceps out of patient as one unit
  - Technician removes needle from suture and patient and helps guide suture through stoma
  - Forceps placed on both ends of suture to prevent accidental movement into the stomach
  - Secure endoscope on table
- Make secure 4 cm loop on cranial end of suture
- Pass loop on PEG tube through suture loop
- Pass other end of PEG tube through PEG loop; pull through completely
  - Lubricate knots and PEG tube liberally
- Technician gently pulls suture through stoma site
- Stoma site carefully incised adjacent to suture when PEG tube reaches stoma site
- Endoscope should follow end of PEG tube through esophagus and visualize correct placement against the stomach wall
  - Observe for blanching of stomach mucosa and excessive bleeding. PEG tube should rotate freely, as shown in Figure 4.14.
- Remove air from stomach post-procedure
- Place bumper over PEG tube near skin

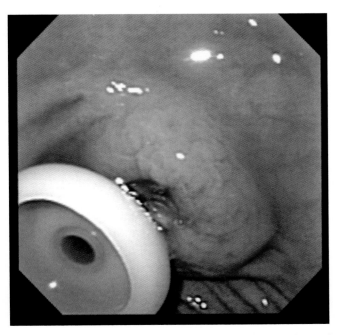

Figure 4.14 PEG tube placed in the antrum. The endoscope is maneuvered near the tube to check for correct placement: no blanching of stomach mucosa should be observed, and the tube can be rotated freely and not tight against the stomach wall.

- Option – cable tie placed *carefully* above the bumper to hold in place (use scissors to cut off excess cable tie; using a cable tie gun will occlude the tube!).
  - Sterile 2 × 2 gauze around the tube at incision
- Draw a line around the tube above bumper
  - Reference point for clients to monitor in case the tube shifts
- Place plastic clamp over PEG tube and secure to middle of tube
  - Keeps food from exiting the tube
- Cut tube to desired length and place feeding adapter on tube end; secure with cable tie
- Stockinette/T-shirt over thoracic limbs and covering PEG tube
  - May be easier to place on patient when awake
- E-collar at all times

SAMPLE COLLECTION AND PROCESSING

The objective for biopsying the GI tract is simple – diagnostic samples – and it starts with good biopsy techniques. Communication is essential between endoscopist and technician, especially if no camera is involved. Keep it simple – create a quiet environment, avoid distractions, and use basic words such as "open" and "close."

GI biopsies usually begin in the duodenum and are performed when retracting the endoscope. One biopsy technique involves turning the insertion tip into the duodenal mucosa, then using endoscope suction to draw the sample into the forceps. The caudal duodenal flexure can also be a good biopsy site. Re-biopsying at the same site (termed "double biting") provides a deeper sample. Eight to ten biopsy samples are recommended from the duodenum. Avoid the duodenal papilla (the pancreatic duct opening) when biopsying. Never biopsy without visualization – it is easy to pass the forceps too far into the duodenum and lose sight of what is biopsied.

Biopsying the stomach should be performed in a systematic manner – seemingly normal-appearing mucosa could be significant histologically. Three or four diagnostic biopsy samples should be taken from each area – pyloral area, antrum, body, and cardia. Avoid biopsies of the pylorus and LES directly. Grossly abnormal areas that are biopsied should be separated from normal-appearing samples. Biopsying around the pylorus can yield smaller biopsies as it is composed of tough smooth muscle. The rugal folds and incisura provide a ridge for the biopsy forceps to bite into for larger samples, as shown in Figures 4.15 and 4.16. A good technique to try is to open the flexible forceps in the stomach and bring the wings back so they are against the endoscope. The endoscopist then pushes the forceps into the mucosa and a biopsy is taken. Biopsying tough esophageal tissue is especially difficult, and will yield very small samples, even using spiked pulmonary biopsy forceps.

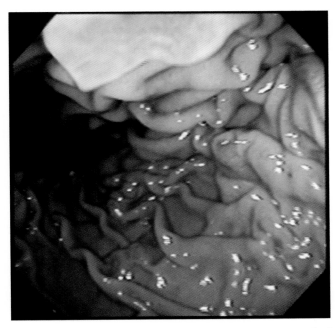

Figure 4.15 Rugal folds in the stomach at time of biopsy. Deflating the stomach slightly reveals an excellent site for biopsy forceps to acquire a diagnostic sample.

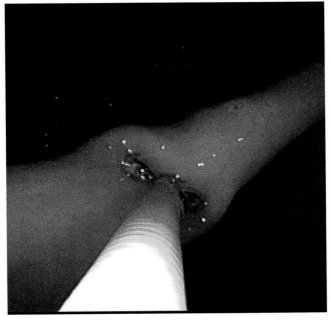

Figure 4.16 The incisura angularis provides a prime area for stomach biopsies. The endoscope can be easily maneuvered to achieve a parallel position for the biopsy forceps. If a retroflex or J-maneuver is used, place the biopsy forceps in the instrument channel first.

To remove the biopsy from the forceps, open the forceps and carefully remove the sample with a 25 Fr needle. If the samples are to be placed on a cassette, it is best to place the samples with the cut end towards the cassette so that the whole villi can be examined when the sample is processed. Cytology slides may be made by touching a biopsy sample on a glass slide several times.

Although not performed routinely, fluid from the duodenum can also be obtained using aspiration tube kits and submitted for culture and/or cytology.

Samples should be labeled with patient identification, number of biopsies, location, endoscopist and date of procedure. GI biopsy samples are placed in formalin unless specified otherwise.

POST-PROCEDURE PATIENT CARE

After the endoscope has been safely removed from the patient, the oral cavity should be examined for esophageal reflux. If present, the esophagus should be suctioned or alternatively lavaged, then the mouth speculum removed. Post-operative pain medication should be considered (see Chapter 3).

COMPLICATIONS

Although rare, perforations of the GI wall could occur from forceful scoping or damaged mucosa, especially around an ulcerated area, esophageal stricture, or foreign body removal site. Gastric overdistension from excessive air insufflation can lead to tachycardia and hypotension with continuing complications if left untreated. Patients should be closely monitored after extubation for gastric dilatation/volvulus. Rupture of major blood vessels can occur during foreign body removal or esophageal balloon dilation.

Endoscope channels can become clogged during an EGD procedure, especially if excessive food is present and suction is used. Immediate post-procedure endoscope flushing should be performed.

SUGGESTED READING

Martin-Flores, M., Scrivani, P.V., Loew, E., Gleed, C.A., and Ludders, J.W. (2014) Maximal and submaximal mouth opening with mouth gags in cats: implications for maxillary artery blood flow. *Vet. J.*, **200**(**1**), 60–64.

Radlinski, M.G. (ed.) (2009) Endoscopy. *Vet. Clin. North Am. Small Anim. Pract.*, **39**(**5**), 817–992.

Tams, T. and Rawlings, C.A. (2011) *Small Animal Endoscopy*, 3rd edn. Elsevier Mosby, St Louis, MO, pp. 41–215.

5 Lower gastrointestinal tract endoscopy

Susan Cox

William R. Pritchard Veterinary Medical Teaching Hospital, University of California-Davis, Davis, California, USA

Colonoscopy visualizes the large intestine, which includes the cecum and ascending, transverse, and descending colon segments and terminates at the rectum and anus. Ileoscopy examines the ileum – the distal portion of the small intestine. Proctoscopy examines the descending colonic segment only. Colonoscopy is usually performed as an adjunct to an esophagogastroduodenoscopy (EGD) procedure, but can also be performed as a solitary procedure based on large bowel clinical signs. Lower gastrointestinal (GI) tract endoscopies are also routinely performed on patients before surgery to determine the exact location and length of a mass lesion. The technician plays a pivotal role in obtaining diagnostic samples, and also in patient preparation.

PATIENT PREPARATION

First, fecal material needs to be evacuated from the patient. A clean colon leads to better visualization, diagnostic samples and preservation of equipment. All patients having lower GI tract endoscopy procedures should be hospitalized the morning before the procedure and food withheld the night before admittance. Dogs are housed in a large enclosure or run. Cats should be placed in a large cage with a litter box accessible at all times.

If proctoscopy is being performed, 2–3 warm water enemas throughout the day before the procedure are adequate at 5–10 mL/kg per dose. A large-diameter (14–18 Fr) red rubber catheter with a catheter-tipped 60 mL syringe works well for cats and small dogs, and disposable enema bags can be used for larger dogs. The lubricated catheter should slide into the colon easily, and the dose is administered as the catheter is slowly pulled back. Hypertonic phosphate enemas are

Endoscopy for the Veterinary Technician, First Edition. Edited by Susan Cox.
© 2016 John Wiley & Sons, Inc. Published 2016 by John Wiley & Sons, Inc.

contraindicated in cats, as they cause hypernatremia and hyperphosphatemia. Additives in many other commercial enema solutions can alter mucosal architecture and should be avoided.

Evacuation of fecal material for colonoscopy/ileoscopy requires the use of oral colonic preparations for a complete lower GI tract examination. Osmoprep® sodium phosphate 1.5 g tablets (Salix Pharmceuticals, Raleigh, NC, USA) have become widely used. A dose of 1 g per 3 kg body weight orally every 4–6 h the day before a procedure is recommended. Since the method of action is to draw fluid from the body and into the colon, water should always be available and intravenous fluid therapy should be considered. Intestinal lavage solutions such as CoLyte® (Alaven Pharmaceutical, Marietta, GA, USA) or GoLYTELY® (Braintree Laboratories, Braintree, MA, USA) can also be used. These preparations contain replacement electrolytes and polyethylene glycol, which acts as an osmotic agent. Solutions are given via a stomach tube in dogs and dosed at 20–30 mL/kg 3–4 times over the 24 h prior to the procedure, and once up to 4 h before the procedure. In cats, a nasoesophageal tube can be placed and the solution given in two doses of 10–20 mL/kg the day before the procedure with a syringe pump. Several warm water enemas may also be given in both cats and dogs the day before and up to 2 h before colonoscopy.

Patients undergoing colonoscopy should be monitored closely for signs of vomition, bloat, gastric torsion, and possible solution aspiration. Cats with nasoesophageal tubes should have an Elizabethan collar placed. Always make sure that the patient has defecated prior to the next dose. Dogs should also be walked on a regular basis.

EQUIPMENT AND INSTRUMENTATION

Flexible endoscopes are used for colonoscopies and rigid sigmoidoscopes (i.e. proctoscopes) can be utilized for proctoscopies. Sigmoidoscope sets are relatively inexpensive and come in several diameters and lengths depending on patient size, as shown in Figure 5.1. In addition to their use in the colon, sigmoidoscopes can also be used for foreign body retrieval in the esophagus. Included in the sigmoidoscope set are an obturator, a bulb insufflator, and a light source attachment, which is shown in Figure 5.2. There are also adapters for use with an otoscope handle as the light source. Disposable plastic sigmoidoscope insertion tubes that attach to a metal base are also available (Welch Allyn, Skaneateles Falls, NY, USA). Uterine or laparoscopic biopsy forceps can be used within the lumen of the sigmoidoscope to obtain larger biopsy samples than with flexible forceps. If excessive fecal material is present, large cotton-tipped applicators known as Scopettes® (Birchwood Laboratories, Eden Prairie, MN, USA) may be used through the opening insertion tube to visualize colonic mucosa.

Flexible GI endoscopes must have working suction and air/water capability and equipped with four-way deflection for easier maneuverability around the

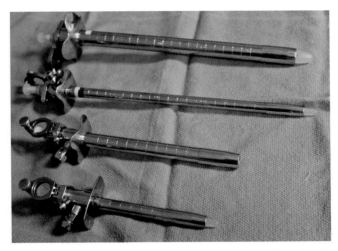

Figure 5.1 Proctoscopes, or sigmoidoscopes, in varying diameters and lengths. The longer 25 cm scopes are also useful for foreign body removal in the esophagus.

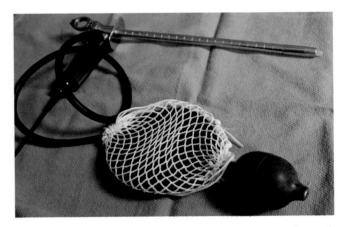

Figure 5.2 19 mm × 25 cm proctoscope with obturator, light source attachment handle, and insufflation bulb.

transverse and descending colon flexures, and to intubate the ileum. A 10 mm o.d. gastroscope with a 2 m working length and a 2.8 mm biopsy channel will be adequate for most medium- and large-sized dogs. For cats and smaller dogs, a 7.9 mm o.d. gastroscope with a 2 mm biopsy channel and 1.4 m working length will be adequate.

If a colonic stricture is encountered, balloon dilation may be indicated. Several sizes of balloon dilators with an optional balloon inflation device to measure radial pressure should be on hand.

Colonoscopy is best performed on a table with a grated surface for easy post-procedure clean-up of the patient and the immediate area. All personnel involved should wear protective gowns, gloves, and shoe covers. Infectious disease protocols should be implemented if a zoonotic disease is suspected.

A complete list of supplies needed for lower GI tract endoscopy is in Box 5.1.

BOX 5.1 EQUIPMENT LIST

- Endoscopes
  - Rigid (sigmoidoscope), with insufflator and light attachment
    - Scopettes
  - Flexible – air/water/suction working, and bowl of water for testing pre- and post-procedure
- Component tower
  - Monitor on
  - Camera or processor and light source
    - Patient info. entered
    - Air/insufflation button depressed
    - Ignition button depressed
      - White balance performed
  - Water bottle and suction attached
  - Image capture
    - Patient info. entered
- Flexible biopsy forceps
- Gowns, examination gloves, shoe covers
- Balloon dilators, ± inflation device with saline for balloon inflation
- Biopsy supplies
  - Biopsy cassettes
  - Formalin jars/culture media
  - Needle for biopsy transfer to cassettes
  - Laboratory forms for biopsy processing
- Lubrication packs/tubes
- Supplies for wrapping tail – gauze wrap, tape
- Stomach tube for relief of abdominal distension
- Endoscopy report to record observations during procedure

PROCEDURES

Colonoscopy/Ileoscopy

- General Anesthesia
  - Uncomfortable procedure
  - Protects endoscope/instrumentation

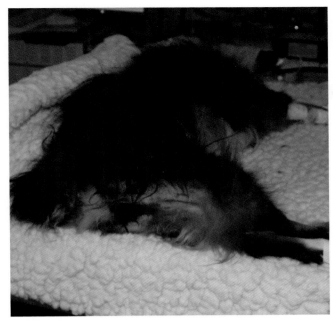

Figure 5.3 Positioning for colonoscopy. The patient is placed in left lateral recumbency. Long tails can be wrapped in gauze and taped cranially.

- Left lateral recumbency, as in Figure 5.3
  - Better visibility
    - Fluid accumulates in the descending colon
- Tail wrapped in stretch gauze and self-adhering bandage material and secured away from the anus
- Digital rectal palpation
  - Palpate anal area for obstructive masses, lesions, perianal hernias, strictures
  - Assess if endoscope will pass safely
- Endoscope into rectum
  - Well-lubricated insertion tip
  - Technician may need to compress the anal area around the endoscope digitally with a gauze square for adequate insufflation to achieve luminal view
- "Slide-by" technique at flexures
  - Descending/transverse and ascending/transverse
    - May briefly lose luminal view
  - Felines – less angular at flexures
- Cecum/ileocolic valve/ileum
  - Cecum appears as a blind pouch

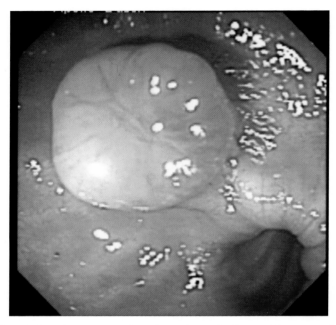

Figure 5.4 Ileocolic junction – rosette-shaped opening to the ileum with cecum adjacent. The cecum should also be explored for masses, etc.

- ▪ Prime area for masses, cecal inversion, intussusception, parasitism
  - ○ Muscular sphincter into ileum (Figure 5.4)
    - ▪ May appear as a slit in cats, rosette-shaped in dogs
    - ▪ If difficult to intubate ileum
      - – Use biopsy forceps as guidewire
        - □ Forceps bite mucosa; guide endoscope through ileocolic valve
      - – If unsuccessful, blind biopsies may be obtained
      - – Be aware that insufflation in the ileum may lead to air accumulation in the stomach; have stomach tube on hand
- • Distal rectum/anus
  - ○ Retroflex view may be attempted in dogs larger than 10 kg.
    - ▪ If biopsying, place biopsy forceps in the channel first before retroflex maneuver, and remove forceps when endoscope is straightened
- • Appearance
  - ○ Grossly normal (as shown in Figure 5.5)
    - ▪ Mucosa should appear smooth, pink, and glistening with vasculature readily seen within the mucosa
    - ▪ Colon should distend readily with insufflation

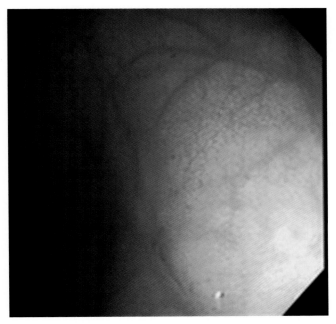

Figure 5.5 Grossly normal colon – colonic mucosa readily apparent, indicating adequate pre-procedure preparation. The mucosa appears smooth and pale pink and easily distends with insufflation. Submucosal vessels are readily visualized.

- ▪ Mucosa should not bleed with endoscope contact
- ▪ Little/no fecal material should be present
- ○ Abnormal Findings
  - ▪ Friable, ulcerative and erosive mucosa
  - ▪ Loss of visualization of submucosal vessels could indicate infiltrative disease.
  - ▪ Polyps, shown in Figure 5.6
  - ▪ Masses such as adenocarcinoma, shown in Figure 5.7, may appear obstructive
- • Colonic stricture encountered
  - ○ Assess
    - ▪ Cause of stricture – neoplasia, etc.
    - ▪ Surgical intervention/balloon dilation
  - ○ Balloon dilation
    - ▪ Dilator alongside endoscope and placed in middle of stricture with endoscopic guidance
    - ▪ Inflate balloon with saline using inflation device
      - – Consult inflation guidelines on dilator packaging

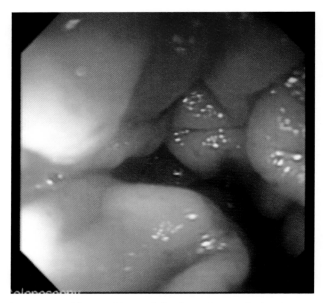

Figure 5.6 Canine presented for vomiting and diarrhea of 1 month duration. Colonoscopy-lumen poorly distended despite insufflation. Lymphoma found with histopathology.

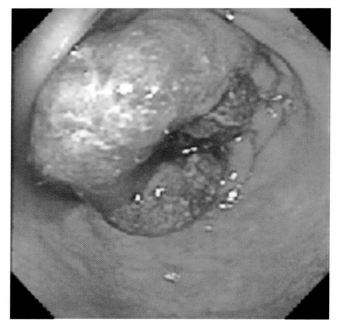

Figure 5.7 Canine presented for hematochezia and large bowel diarrhea. Intraoperative colonoscopy performed, and an obstructive mass was identified and resected. Pathologic diagnosis: adenocarcinoma.

      – Observe for mucosal bleeding, tearing, perforation
      – Several sizes may be used as stricture is reduced
* Biopsies
  ○ Taken retrograde (see Sample collection and processing)
* Encourage endoscopist to complete report

Rigid Proctoscopy

* Examination of the descending colon only
* Heavy sedation or general anesthesia
* Sternal or right lateral recumbency as in Figure 5.8
* Digital rectal examination performed
  ○ Masses, obstructive lesions, perianal hernias may be palpated
* Sigmoidoscope with obturator carefully passed through rectum and into colon
  ○ Well lubricated
* Obturator removed
* Glass window screwed into place
* Bulb insufflator attached to scope
* Colon insufflated
  ○ Technician may need to compress around anus digitally for adequate insufflation/luminal view

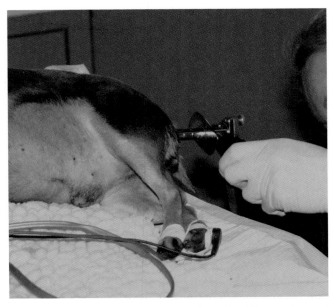

Figure 5.8 Positioning for proctoscopy. Patient is positioned in right lateral recumbency with the hind end toward the end of the table.

○ Biopsy sites visually identified and biopsies obtained
○ Use centimeter measurements on proctoscope to document mass location
• Encourage endoscopist to complete endoscopy report
• Bedside endoscope cleaning

SAMPLE COLLECTION AND PROCESSING

Collection of biopsy samples in colonoscopy is similar to that in an EGD procedure. If intubation of the ileum is unsuccessful, biopsies can be performed blind.
The endoscopist should maneuver the endoscope for a straight-on view of the
ileocolic valve. The closed forceps can then slide through the valve and biopsies can be performed. Colonic flexures allow mucosa to be perpendicular to
the biopsy forceps, and are ideal sites for diagnostic samples. If excessive fecal
material is present, double biting may be necessary to obtain a representative
sample. Biopsy sampling using a proctoscope can provide larger samples of the
distal colon since large-diameter forceps can pass through the wide diameter of
the proctoscope. Proctoscopic biopsies with flexible forceps require the endoscopist to hold the forceps within the proctoscope while the technician operates
them. Once a biopsy site is identified, the forceps are curved onto the mucosa
and the biopsy is taken. A slight tug on the forceps may occur when biopsying
and is normal. Biopsies using rigid forceps should be performed with caution,
since the larger cup area could perforate diseased/necrotic colonic mucosa and
require surgical intervention.

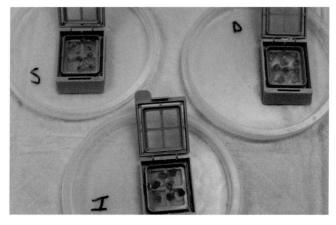

Figure 5.9 Biopsy cassettes with biopsies separated according to location. Each labeled cassette
will be placed in a separate labeled biopsy jar in formalin.

Biopsies of the ileum should be placed separate from colonic biopsies, and masses/lesions encountered in the colon should be placed in a separate cassette/formalin jar from grossly normal colonic biopsies. Figure 5.9 displays biopsy samples from EGD and colonoscopy procedures.

Owing to the nature of the biopsy forceps, endoscopic colonic biopsies sample only the first two layers of the colon – mucosa and submucosa. It is important to place the biopsy samples on the cassette so that the submucosal layer is toward the cassette. When the samples are processed, the slide will contain both mucosal layers.

POST-PROCEDURE PATIENT CARE

Have a stomach tube available to remove air and residual colonic solution from the stomach following ileoscopy. Examine the oral cavity for any regurgitation – suction or gauze squares may be needed to remove the material. Clean and towel-dry the perianal area prior to extubation. Maintaining the tail wrap will help keep the patient comfortable after the procedure – diarrhea and gas accumulation are common outcomes. Clients should be notified that hematochezia is expected after lower GI tract endoscopy, and could continue for 24–48 h.

COMPLICATIONS

Aspiration, bloat, vomition, and gastric torsion could occur from administration of colonic lavage solution. Patients prepared for colonoscopy should be in a run (dogs) or large cage with a litter box (cats) and constantly monitored.

Insufflation of the ileum from the endoscopy could cause air to accumulate in the stomach during the procedure. A stomach tube may be used to remove the air.

Perforation or hemorrhage of the colon from biopsy of diseased mucosa is rare, but should be considered.

SUGGESTED READING

Atkins, C.E., Tyler, R., and Greenlee, P. (1985) Clinical, biochemical, acid–base, and electrolyte abnormalities in cats after hypertonic sodium phosphate enema administration *Am J. Vet. Res.*, **46**(**4**), 980–988.

Lieb, M., Baechtel, M., and Monroe, W. (2004) Complications associated with 355 flexible colonoscopic procedures in dogs. *J. Vet. Intern. Med.*, **18**(**5**), 642–646.

Richter, K.P. and Cleveland, M. (1989) Comparison of an orally administered gastrointestinal lavage solution with traditional enema administration as preparation for colonoscopy in dogs. *J. Am. Vet. Med. Assoc.*, **195**(**12**), 1727–1731.

Tams, T. and Rawlings, C.A. (2011) *Small Animal Endoscopy*, 3rd edn. Elsevier Mosby, St Louis, MO, pp. 217–232.

Willard, M. (2001) Colonoscopy, proctoscopy and ileoscopy. *Vet. Clin. North Am. Small Anim. Pract.*, **31**, 657–669.

6 Upper airway endoscopy

Susan Cox

William R. Pritchard Veterinary Medical Teaching Hospital, University of California-Davis, Davis, California, USA

Thorough upper airway endoscopy (UAE) includes the right and left nasal cavities (rhinoscopy), the nasopharynx (nasopharyngoscopy), the larynx (laryngoscopy), and the oral cavity. If indicated from the pre-endoscopic workup, a computed tomography (CT) scan or radiographs could be helpful in pinpointing the location of a lesion/mass so that diagnostic biopsies can be precise, and to evaluate the cribriform plate. Depending on clinical signs, a laryngoscopy may be performed without a rhinoscopy, or a tracheoscopy/lower airway examination may be added if altered disease processes are found when performing the procedure. It is important to have all the equipment and required personnel assembled with a minimum of outside distractions in case a respiratory emergency occurs.

Discuss the procedure with the endoscopist and have a general plan in place. A laryngeal examination may be necessary to assess laryngeal function, and must be performed before intubation under a light plane of anesthesia (see Chapter 3). Laryngeal biopsies are best performed with the endotracheal tube in place in case bleeding occurs. Nasopharyngoscopy can then be performed before rhinoscopy so that structures can be adequately visualized.

PATIENT PREPARATION

Other than routine anesthetic fasting, no special pre-procedure patient preparation is required for UAE. General anesthesia is required for upper airway examinations. For upper airway procedures, the patient should be placed in sternal recumbency, as shown in Figure 6.1. A rolled-up towel or bolster is placed under the jaw to elevate the head, and two mouth speculae are used on the upper and lower canines to protect the instruments. The mouth speculae can be removed prior to rostral rhinoscopy.

Endoscopy for the Veterinary Technician, First Edition. Edited by Susan Cox.
© 2016 John Wiley & Sons, Inc. Published 2016 by John Wiley & Sons, Inc.

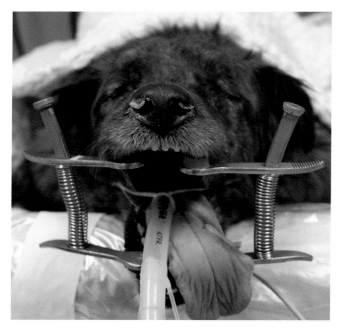

Figure 6.1 Sternal positioning for upper airway examination, with two mouth gags in place on the upper and lower canine teeth.

Infraorbital blocks can help with pain management during and after the procedure. The blocks can be done after anesthesia induction. A "how-to" guide can be found in Chapter 3.

Additionally, moistened lap pads or a gauze pack are placed at the back of the oral cavity prior to rostral rhinoscopy to absorb excess fluids exiting from the nasopharynx. This pack should be checked periodically and replaced if necessary. A labeled piece of tape on the patient's forehead or a colorful string around the pack and exiting the mouth are visual reminders to remove the pack prior to extubation. Absorbent pads or towels should be placed on the floor for easier post-procedure cleaning.

EQUIPMENT AND INSTRUMENTATION

Both rigid and flexible endoscopes are utilized in upper airway procedures. Rigid telescopes are needed to visualize the laryngeal area and rostral nasal cavities. Commercially available rigid rhinoscopes measure 2.7 mm o.d. and 18.5 cm in length with 0° or 30° viewing angles, as shown in Figure 6.2. For rostral rhinoscopy, the instrument sheath can be placed over the telescope and include

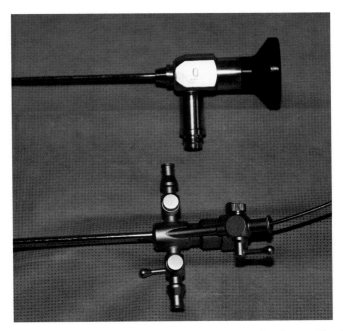

Figure 6.2 A rigid telescope with light cable attachment is pictured at the top. The sheath (also pictured) fits over the telescope and locks in place at the base. Ports to attach saline infusion and suction/drainage extend out from the side and can be opened/closed with levers. The instrument channel is positioned dorsally.

ports for flush, suction attachments, and a 2.0 mm instrument port for 1.8 mm instruments. Adding the sheath increases the telescope's o.d. to 17.5 Fr, which may be too large to fit into the nasal cavities of smaller dogs and most cats. If flushing is needed, a 3.5–8 Fr red rubber catheter with saline-filled syringes can be placed alongside the telescope. The gauze pack should be checked and replaced as needed if copious flushing is used.

Flexible endoscopes are used for nasopharyngoscopy and can be utilized for rostral rhinoscopy, especially if the frontal sinus can be accessed (sinuscopy). An o.d. of 5–5.3 mm with a 2.0 mm operating channel is an ideal size for canine or feline patients, especially when retroflexing behind the soft palate to observe the nasopharynx. Any foreign bodies can be removed as soon as they are visualized with flexible biopsy forceps passed through the biopsy/suction channel. Alligator-type rigid forceps can also be passed alongside the telescope in the nasal cavity for visual retrieval of foreign objects such as plant awns or seeds. Rigid cup biopsy forceps such as those shown in Figure 6.3 are available in 2, 3, and 4 mm cup sizes for biopsies of the rostral nasal cavity and laryngeal masses/lesions. These forceps can become dull over time and should be sharpened as needed.

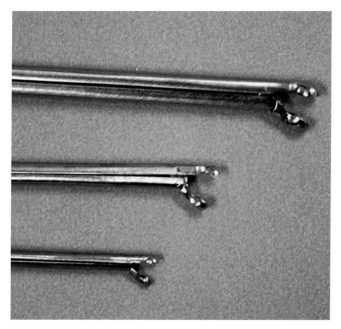

Figure 6.3 Cup biopsy forceps in 2, 3, and 4 mm biopsy cup sizes. These rigid forceps are used alongside the telescope when a specific location must be visually biopsied. Depending upon use, the cups should be sharpened on a regular basis.

A full list of equipment needed to perform a diagnostic upper airway examination is listed in Box 6.1.

PROCEDURE

- Observe laryngeal function prior to intubation
  - Assess vocal folds abducting properly
    - Light anesthetic plane
      - Full, deep breaths needed to evaluate properly
      - Team member observes chest excursions and tells endoscopist when patient inspires
      - Dopamine hydrochloride on hand to facilitate deeper, even breathing
      - See Chapter 3 for protocol
    - Visual observation with laryngoscope or rigid telescope for group participation
    - Brief proximal tracheoscopy with rigid telescope if indicated
  - Endotracheal intubation

BOX 6.1 EQUIPMENT FOR A DIAGNOSTIC UPPER AIRWAY ENDOSCOPIC EXAMINATION

- Endoscope
  - Flexible – nasopharyngoscopy/rostral rhinoscopy
  - Rigid, ± sheath – laryngoscopy/rostral rhinoscopy
- Component tower
  - Monitor on
  - Camera/processor and light source
    - Patient info. entered
    - Ignition button depressed-light source
      - White balance performed
    - Optional suction attachment
      - At control section on smaller diameter endoscopes
  - Image capture
    - Patient info. entered
- Biopsy instruments
  - Flexible forceps
  - Rigid cup forceps – 2, 3, or 4 mm cup size
- Alligator-type rigid foreign body retrieval forceps
- Mouth speculae ×2
- Infraorbital blocks – see Chapter 3
- Bolster/sandbag for headrest
- 0.9% saline flush
  - 1 L bag of 0.9% saline in ice–water bath if excessive bleeding
  - Syringes
  - 3.5–8 Fr red rubber catheter
- Lap pads
- Lidocaine jelly
- Oxymetazoline drops for vasoconstriction
- Non-bacteriostatic lube packs
- Ice packs
- Cotton-tipped applicators
- Biopsy supplies
  - Cassettes ×3 – right nasal cavity, left nasal cavity, nasopharynx
  - Biopsy jars labeled with patient information
  - Laboratory submission form
- Endoscopy report to record observations during procedure

- Laryngoscopy
  - Both sides symmetric
    - Note mucosal color, excessive mucus, edema/inflammation
    - Biopsy if indicated
- Oral examination
  - Sweep tonsils for foreign objects, check under tongue, palpate soft palate

- Nasopharyngoscopy
  - ◦ Anatomy
    - ▪ Choanae – bilateral openings to nasal cavity, separated by vomer bone
  - ◦ Tongue pulled cranially, neck extended
  - ◦ Flexible endoscope into oral cavity and flexed above soft palate
    - ▪ Highly stimulating to patient – may need to pause until deeper plane of anesthesia achieved
      - – Apply lidocaine gel to oropharynx to facilitate retroflex
    - ▪ Image on monitor inversed – up/down, left/right
    - ▪ Standard appearance, as shown in Figure 6.4
      - – Pale pink in color
      - – Sub-mucosal vessels apparent
      - – Choanae can appear dark or turbinates seen in brachycephalic patients
    - ▪ Note foreign bodies, mucosal color, masses (see Figure 6.5), stenosis
      - – Remove foreign bodies at first sign
      - – Watch for polyps in felines
    - ▪ Biopsy/retrieval
      - – Pass the biopsy forceps into channel before flexing endoscope

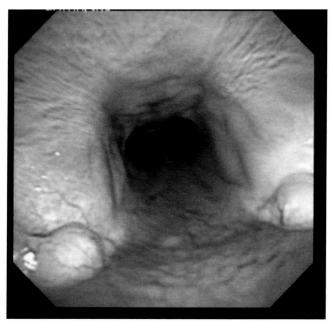

Figure 6.4 Grossly normal nasopharynx in a dog. Patient is positioned as in Figure 6.1. Soft palate is ventral, and the left side of the image is the dog's right side. The choanae (dark areas) connect the nasal passages to the nasopharynx.

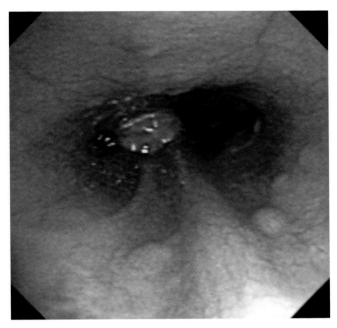

Figure 6.5 A mass in the right choana of a dog. Biopsies were taken with flexible biopsy forceps through a flexible endoscope. The forceps were fed through the biopsy channel before flexing the endoscope into the nasopharynx. Histopathology revealed osteosarcoma.

  □ Saves wear and tear on channel
 – Assistant extends forceps and takes biopsy
  □ Relax bend in the endoscope after the biopsy has been taken and before removing the forceps to avoid perforating the channel
 – Check back of oral cavity for excessive bleeding
- Rostral rhinoscopy
  ○ Flexible endoscope can be used if:
   ▪ Appropriate size for nasal cavity
   ▪ Frontal sinus can be accessed
  ○ Moistened lap pad or gauze packs placed in caudal oral cavity to catch residual fluid
   ▪ Check endotracheal tube cuff for adequate inflation
  ○ Measure rigid scope from medial canthus to end of nose, as shown in Figure 6.6 – mark with tape
   ▪ Alerts endoscopist to site of cribriform plate, a thin bone between the brain and nasal cavity
    – Can be compromised in fungal diseases, neoplasia
  ○ Unaffected nasal cavity entered first, if known, then affected side

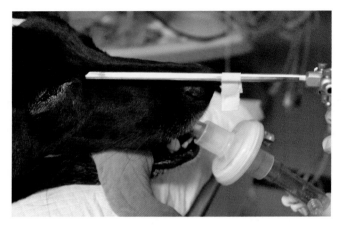

Figure 6.6 Measurement taken from the end of the nose to the medial canthus with rigid telescope and marked with tape. This mark reminds the endoscopist of how far the rhinoscope can go before the cribriform plate is reached. Figure 6.11 shows both the telescope and biopsy forceps similarly labeled.

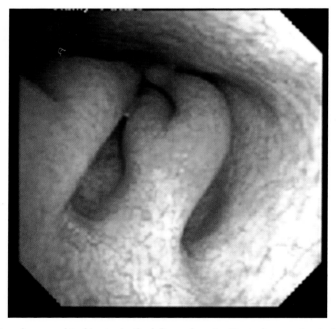

Figure 6.7 Grossly normal turbinates in the left nasal cavity. Normal-appearing turbinates are tightly packed together and pale pink in color.

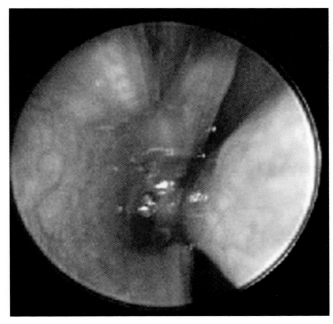

Figure 6.8 Plant awn in the nasal cavity. Removal is best achieved with visualization and rigid alligator forceps alongside the telescope or flexible biopsy forceps through the sheath.

- Standard appearance, as in Figure 6.7
  - Nasal cavity divided into ventral, middle and dorsal meati
  - Turbinates packed together
  - Pale pink in color
  - Minimal fluid present (fluid should be clear)
  ○ Inspect ventral aspect first, since turbinates are friable, then work upwards
    - Note foreign bodies as shown in Figure 6.8 (remove at first sign), masses (see Figure 6.9), mucosal color (hyperemia), turbinate architecture/absence, fungal plaques (see Figure 6.10)
    - If sinus involvement (neoplasia, fungal disease), sinuscopy or nasal trephination may be needed
    - Suction/saline flush indicated if visualization lost
      - Cold 0.9% saline flush or oxymetazoline drops instilled into both nasal cavities causes vasoconstriction
        □ Do not use if cribriform plate compromised
      - Flushing extraneous mucoid material can be therapeutic
  ○ Biopsies performed after nasal cavities viewed
    - Visualized biopsies best

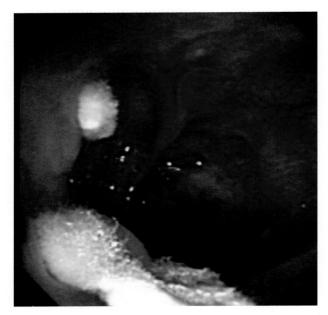

Figure 6.9 *Aspergillus* sp. in the nasal cavity with frontal sinus in the background. This fungus can appear as white to yellow filamentous plaques and cause destruction of the cribriform plate, nasal septum, and turbinates.

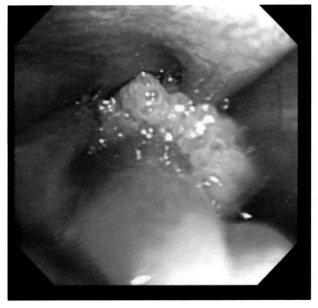

Figure 6.10 Polypoid carcinoma found in both nasal cavities of a dog. Note the difference in color and texture with the surrounding turbinates. Visual biopsies, as in Figure 6.11, give the best chance of a correct diagnosis.

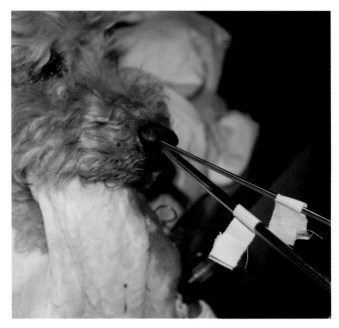

Figure 6.11 Visual biopsy of the right nasal cavity. The sheathed telescope is passed first, and the affected area is visualized. The biopsy forceps are then passed alongside the telescope, and the biopsy is taken.

- – Flexible forceps through sheath
  - ▫ Open forceps only when wings can be visualized
- – Rigid forceps alongside telescope, as in Figure 6.11
- ○ Remove lap sponge/gauze pack when procedure complete
  - ■ Examine oral cavity for excessive fluid accumulation – use suction, cotton-tipped applicators
  - ■ If dental disease suspected, dental probing can be performed
    - – Position in ventro-dorsal
  - ■ Ice pack on nose if excessively bleeding; delay recovery until active bleeding stops
- ○ Encourage endoscopist to complete endoscopy report

SAMPLE COLLECTION AND PROCESSING

Biopsies of the upper airway can be challenging, mainly due to the friability of nasal mucosa and subsequent loss of visualization, especially in the nasal cavity. It is essential to obtain visualized biopsies from mass lesions first. If bleeding occurs, copious 0.9% cold saline flushes or waiting until the bleeding stops can provide better odds for a diagnostic sample. Impression smears may be made from collected samples for immediate cytologic evaluation before being placed in formalin. Smaller samples are then placed in biopsy cassettes and labeled appropriately. Separate cassettes/formalin jars can be used for biopsies of suspected lesions/masses.

For fungal culture/identification submittal, direct visualization of the biopsied specimen is favored over blind or brush sampling. Suspected fungal samples should be submitted in a separate cassette and an additional sample placed in a sterile container, such as a red-topped tube (RTT), or check with your reference laboratory for their recommendations.

POST-PROCEDURE PATIENT CARE

As the endotracheal tube is being removed, leave the cuff partially inflated so that any residual fluid will be moved out of the trachea. Patients recovering from UAE procedures should be placed in an observation cage that is away from excessive traffic. Many of these patients have bloody discharge and sneezing episodes, so it is best to have a clear area around the cage. A slow recovery would be optimum for these patients – see Chapter 3 for guidelines.

COMPLICATIONS

Bleeding or epistaxis is expected during and after an upper airway procedure. Patients should be kept in the hospital overnight and monitored, especially if excessive bleeding is observed. Clients should be notified that epistaxis could be expected for at least 5–7 days after discharge from the hospital. Aspiration pneumonia can also occur from excessive fluid drainage, so careful monitoring of excessive fluid build-up in the oropharynx is essential. Inflammation of laryngeal tissue could also occur from excessive manipulation and may require medical management. If the cribriform plate is not intact, encephalitis could occur and require immediate intervention.

SUGGESTED READING

DiLorenzi, D., Bonfanti, U., Masserdotti, C., Caldin, M., and Furlanello, T. (2006) Diagnosis of canine aspergillosis from cytological examination; an evaluation of 4 different collection techniques. *J. Small Anim. Pract.* 2006, **47**(**6**), 316–319.

Johnson, L.R. (2010) *Clinical Canine and Feline Respiratory Medicine.* Blackwell Publishing, Ames, IA, pp. 20–27.

Tams, T. and Rawlings, C.A. (2011) *Small Animal Endoscopy*, 3rd edn. Elsevier Mosby, St Louis, MO, pp. 563–577.

7 Lower airway endoscopy

Susan Cox

William R. Pritchard Veterinary Medical Teaching Hospital, University of California-Davis, Davis, California, USA

Lower airway endoscopy (LAE) starts with an examination of the trachea (tracheoscopy) and continues with visualization of the airways (bronchoscopy). It is an invasive, critical procedure involving patients that are often struggling to breathe. As a result, LAE procedures should be as well organized as possible to limit anesthesia time. It is recommended that this procedure be a team effort, with qualified personnel designated to a single task. For example, one team member should be assigned to anesthesia induction and monitoring and another to monitoring endoscopy equipment. This approach allows the endoscopist to concentrate solely on the patient, and perform the procedure efficiently.

An advantage of bronchoscopy is that although it is a short procedure, it is a means of obtaining diagnostic information in a short amount of time. Cytology and culture of bronchoalveolar lavage (BAL) fluid and locating sites of masses or foreign bodies can aid significantly in diagnosis and treatment. Bronchoscopy can also be performed intraoperatively in conjunction with a thoracotomy, or with fluoroscopic guidance for tracheal stent placement.

PATIENT PREPARATION

General anesthesia is required for all LAE procedures, so routine patient fasting is required. Oxygen should be administered via facemask for at least 10 min prior to induction, and be nearby if laryngeal function is being assessed. The patient is positioned in sternal recumbency with the head resting on a towel roll or a sandbag, as shown in Figure 7.1.

Endoscopy for the Veterinary Technician, First Edition. Edited by Susan Cox.
© 2016 John Wiley & Sons, Inc. Published 2016 by John Wiley & Sons, Inc.

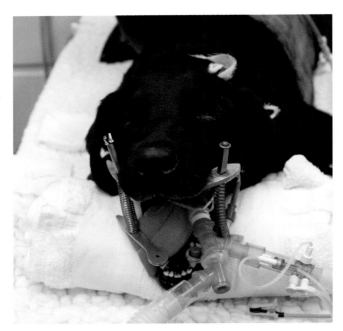

Figure 7.1 Patient positioning for lower airway endoscopy. The dog is positioned in sternal recumbency. Two mouth speculae are used to protect the endoscope. The short endotracheal tube can be secured behind the head or on top of the nose. A close-up of bronchoscopy adapter is seen in Figure 7.2.

EQUIPMENT AND INSTRUMENTATION

Flexible endoscopes are primarily used for LAE, although rigid telescopes may be used to view the proximal trachea. Most bronchoscopes have two-way deflection (up/down), although smaller diameter gastroscopes with four-way deflection can be used in larger dogs. Urethroscopes (2.9 mm o.d. × 100 cm) used in cystoscopies in male dogs can be used for smaller canines and felines and should have an instrument channel for performing BAL and foreign body retrieval. The most common size for bronchoscopes in the cat and small dog is 5–5.5 cm o.d. with a 55 cm working length and a 1.2 cm instrument channel. Larger dogs (>25 kg) require at least 90 cm working length and a 2.0 cm instrument channel for 1.8 mm instruments. When purchasing a bronchoscope, look for a model with an instrument channel port that snugly fits a syringe hub. This feature creates a better seal for maximum BAL retrieval.

Suction and air/water functions should not be used in bronchoscopy. Inadvertently insufflating in a small airway could cause a ballooning effect distally, and suction could damage or tear delicate lung mucosa.

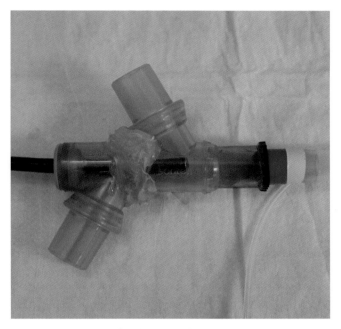

Figure 7.2 Two Sontek adapters are fused to allow for oxygen and inhalation gas delivery with gas scavenge as the endoscope is passed through the endotracheal tube. Two flexible membranes are also included within the adapter.

Oxygen delivery can be accomplished using a variety of methods. For larger dogs that can tolerate a 7.5 Fr or greater endotracheal tube, a customized endotracheal adapter (Sontek Medical, Hingham, MA, USA), as shown in Figure 7.2, can be attached to a short endotracheal tube (Surgivet, Dublin, OH, USA) placed just beyond the larynx. Ports on the sides of the adapter attach anesthetic gas and CO_2 scavenge. The endoscope passes through the adapter and the tube and into the trachea. This arrangement allows the endoscopist a broader view of the trachea while allowing oxygen/gas inhalation delivery. Anesthesia adapters should not be used in endoscopes smaller than 6 mm o.d. because of possible endoscope damage. For smaller dogs and cats, jet ventilation through a large-bore (14–16 mm) catheter alongside the endoscope with injectable anesthetic constant-rate infusion works well, and is discussed further in Chapter 3. Oxygen through the biopsy channel can also be adapted, although this can be inadequate with passage of instruments or BAL fluid.

Pulmonary biopsy forceps have a fenestrated cup with a spike in the center to biopsy tough bronchial tissue. Always make sure that the end of the forceps is out of the biopsy channel when deploying. Foreign bodies may be retrieved with cupped biopsy forceps.

BALs are performed with a predetermined amount, using warmed 0.9% saline in a 20 mL syringe. Several prefilled syringes should be prepared before the procedure begins. Application of lubrication on the outside of the endoscope should be minimal, as it can interfere with cytologic analysis. Cotton-tipped applicators can be useful for cleaning debris from the adapter before the endoscope is reinserted.

Strictures of the tracheal lumen are rare, and often require immediate intervention. Small-diameter balloons with an inflation device should be available.

A complete list of supplies is listed in Box 7.1.

BOX 7.1 EQUIPMENT FOR A LOWER AIRWAY ENDOSCOPIC EXAMINATION.

- Appropriate endoscope
  - Rigid telescope if laryngoscopy also performed
  - Flexible endoscope
  - Oxygen/anesthetic delivery system
    - Jet ventilator
    - Oxygen adapted for biopsy channel
    - Airway adapter
- Component tower
  - Monitor on
  - Camera/light source/processor
    - Patient info. entered
    - Insufflation off
    - Suction/water bottle not used
    - Ignition/light on
      - White balance
  - Image capture
    - Patient info entered
- Mouth speculae ×2
- Foreign body retrieval forceps
- Pulmonary biopsy forceps
- BAL supplies
  - Non-bacteriostatic 0.9% saline
  - 20 mL syringes
  - Option – suction trap
- Balloon dilators with inflation device
- Biopsy supplies
  - Tissue cassettes
  - Formalin jars
  - RTT/Culturette for sterile sample
- Non-bacteriostatic lube packets
- 0.9% saline-soaked gauze
- Laboratory submittal forms
- Endoscopy report for recording observations during procedure

---

PROCEDURE

- Preoxygenate
  - 10 min via facemask
  - All team members assembled and focused on procedure
  - Endoscope/telescope ready
- Laryngeal function assessed prior to intubation
  - Light anesthesia plane
  - Arytenoid motion evaluated as patient breathes
  - Doxapram IV can be used as respiratory stimulant (see Chapter 3)
  - Intubation/O_2 catheter placement
- Brief oropharyngeal examination
  - Two mouth speculae on right/left upper and lower canines
  - Examine tonsils (see Figure 7.3)
    - In/out of tonsilar crypts, inflammation, foreign objects
  - Palpate soft/hard palate
  - Look under/around tongue
- Tracheoscopy
  - Lightly lubricate around distal insertion tip of endoscope
    - Excessive lubrication can interfere with cytology findings

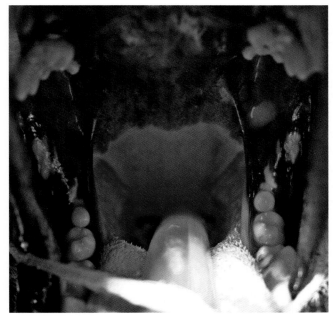

Figure 7.3 Oral examination in a large dog in sternal recumbency. Note the tonsils are within the tonsilar crypts. The soft palate can also be easily palpated, and the tongue can be moved and searched for masses, foreign bodies, etc.

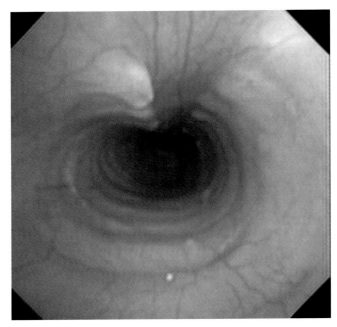

Figure 7.4 A grossly normal trachea in a dog. The mucosa is pale pink, and the dorsal tracheal membrane is dorsal in the image.

- Assistant may need to extend tongue cranially for endoscope intubation
- Dorsal membrane kept dorsal
- Standard appearance – see Figure 7.4
  - Round tube-like structure
  - Pale pink in color
  - Vasculature slightly visible
- Observations
  - Tracheal collapse
    - Mainly seen in small-breed dogs
    - Assess and record severity:
      - Grade 1 – 25% collapse from normal
      - Grade 2 – 50%
      - Grade 3 – 75%, as shown in Figure 7.5
      - Grade 4 – 100%
  - Mucosal color – pale pink is standard
  - Masses, strictures, foreign objects, as shown in Figures 7.6 and 7.7
    - Remove/biopsy at first sign
    - Ballooning strictures may be indicated
  - Presence of fluid
    - Record amount, clarity

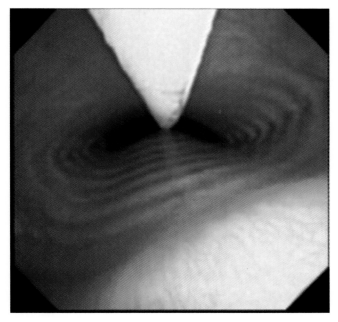

Figure 7.5 Tracheal collapse in a dog. The dorsal tracheal membrane is dorsal in the image, and the dog is in sternal recumbency. The white jet ventilator catheter is also present. Tracheal collapse was scored as Grade 3 (75%). Bronchial airway collapse in this patient is also depicted in Figure 7.9.

- ○ Carina
  - ▪ Separates right and left main bronchi
  - ▪ Assess for symmetry, masses, fluid accumulation
- • Bronchoscopy
  - ○ Systematic approach
    - ▪ Enlarge diagrams in Figures 7.8 and 7.9, attach to monitor, and use as reference
  - ○ Image reversed – right side is on the left on monitor
  - ○ Observations
    - ▪ Standard appearance, as shown in Figure 7.10
      - – Mucosa should be pale pink in color
      - – Minimal secretions present
      - – Rounded airways
      - – Vasculature readily seen
    - ▪ Abnormal
      - – Airway dilation, also termed bronchiectasis, as shown in Figure 7.11
      - – Airway collapse, identified as bronchomalacia, depicted in Figure 7.12
        - ▫ Note severity in percentages in record

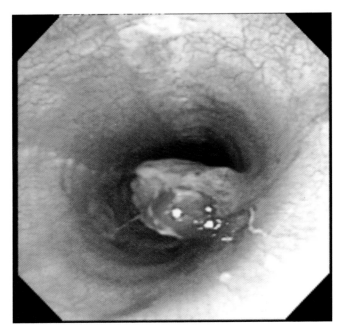

Figure 7.6 Caudal tracheal mass in a dog. The patient is presented in sternal recumbency with the dorsal tracheal membrane dorsal. A laser-capable endoscope was used with a diode laser to debulk mass. Histopathology revealed a benign mass.

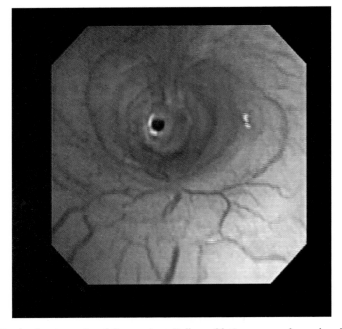

Figure 7.7 Tracheal stricture in a feline patient. Balloon dilation was performed and multiple recheck bronchoscopies were carried out with great success.

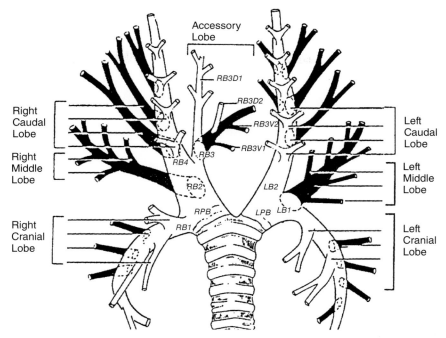

Figure 7.8 Diagrammatic representation of canine bronchial tree. It is suggested to copy and resize to use as a reference when performing bronchoscopy. Source: reprinted with permission from Amis, T.C. and McKieman, B.C. (1986) Systematic identification of endobronchial anatomy during bronchoscopy. *Am. J. Vet. Res.*, 1986, **47**(**12**), 2649–2657.

- Masses/foreign objects
  □ Remove at first sign
- Purulent material, as shown in Figure 7.13
- Fluid accumulation
- Hyperemic mucosa
- Parasites
○ Assess airways for BAL sites
○ Remove endoscope
  ▪ Flush biopsy channel – sterile 0.9% saline, then air
  ▪ Wipe down insertion tube – saline-soaked gauze sponges
  ▪ Clean adapter membranes
○ Careful re-entry for BALs, brush cytology
  ▪ Avoid mucosal contamination
○ BAL
  ▪ Instill a predetermined amount of sterile non-bacteriostatic 0.9% saline through biopsy channel into wedged airway using 20 mL syringes
  ▪ Clear channel with 3–5 mL of air
  ▪ Gently aspirate fluid back into syringe
    - Suction trap attached to biopsy channel optional

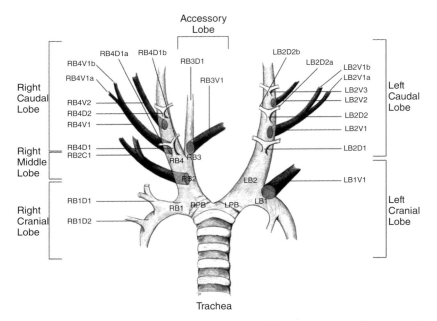

Figure 7.9 Diagrammatic representation of feline bronchial tree. It is suggested to copy and resize to use as a reference when performing bronchoscopy. Source: Caccamo, R., Twedt, D.C., Buracco, P., and McKiernan, B.C. (2007) Endoscopic bronchial anatomy in the cat. *J. Feline Med. Surg.*, **9(2)**, 10. Copyright © 2007. Reprinted with permission of Sage.

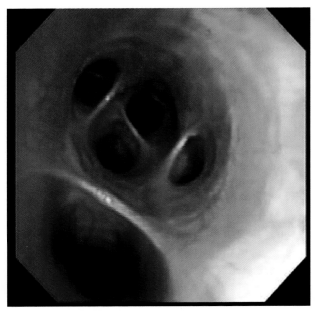

Figure 7.10 Normal lung field in a canine patient. Mucosa is light pink, airways are rounded, and minimal secretions are present.

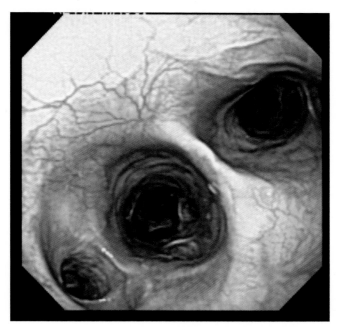

Figure 7.11 Bronchiectasis in a canine. Proximal airway openings are enlarged, usually due to chronic inflammation. Increased vascularity of lung mucosa should also be noted.

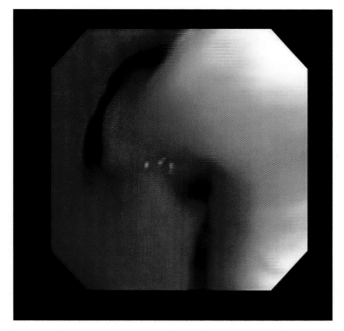

Figure 7.12 Airway collapse in a dog (see also Figure 7.4). Also termed bronchomalacia.

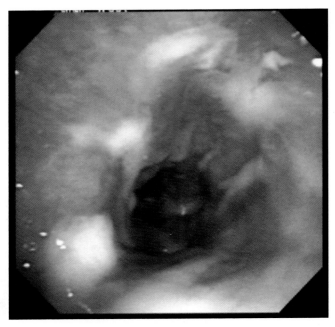

Figure 7.13 Mucus accumulation in the lung of a dog. The location should be noted at first pass and a BAL performed in this area. Prior to performing BAL, the endoscope should be removed from the patient, wiped down with saline-soaked gauze, and the instrument channel flushed with saline.

- ■ Inform endoscopist if negative pressure felt with syringe
- ■ Retrieved fluid should have layer of foam (surfactant) – confirms contact with alveolar space, as shown in Figure 7.14
- ○ Probe teeth if warranted
- Encourage endoscopist to complete report

SAMPLE COLLECTION AND PROCESSING

Each BAL sample should be labeled with patient information and retrieval site. Samples for culture can be pooled – several drops of each sample are placed in a sterile red-topped tube (RTT) for submittal. Biopsies are placed in sample cassettes and formalin. Guarded brush cytology samples can be submitted in their original packaging, or the brush end can be cut off and placed in an RTT.

POST PROCEDURE PATIENT CARE

Patients that are jet ventilated or catheters used for oxygen delivery can be either intubated with a standard endotracheal tube and oxygenated until awake, or

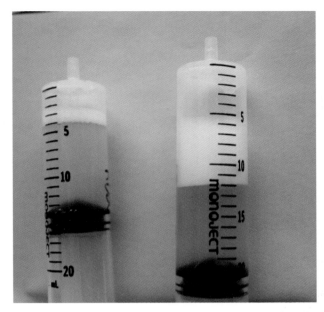

Figure 7.14 BAL samples. The surfactant (white foam) seen at the top of the fluid in the syringes signifies effective contact with the alveolar space.

flow-by oxygen used with mask post-extubation if tolerated. An oxygen cage may be needed for critical patients following the procedure. Refer to Chapter 3 for additional information.

COMPLICATIONS

Coughing or increased airway obstruction with accompanying stress from the procedure can warrant careful monitoring of these patients. Oxygen, endotracheal tubes, and a laryngoscope should be readily available until the patient is ambulatory.

SUGGESTED READING

Johnson, L.R. (2010) *Clinical Canine and Feline Respiratory Medicine*. Blackwell Publishing, Ames, IA, pp. 27–37.
Tams, T. and Rawlings, C.A. (2011) *Small Animal Endoscopy*, 3rd edn. Elsevier Mosby, St Louis, MO, pp. 339–359.

8   Urogenital endoscopy

Susan Cox
*William R. Pritchard Veterinary Medical Teaching Hospital, University
of California–Davis, Davis, California, USA*

Cystoscopy had not received much attention in clinical practice until the recent development of smaller diameter endoscopes and instrumentation, as a result of which equipment has become more cost-effective and is adaptable for other procedures such as rhinoscopy and laryngoscopy. Residents are being trained in cystoscopy at teaching hospitals and are capable of performing this procedure in private practice for a growing clientele. They will need technical assistance, technicians who know how to operate and troubleshoot the equipment before and during the procedure, and to document findings for the endoscopist.

Cystoscopy is defined as the visualization of the vagina, urethral opening, urethra, bladder, and ureteral openings. Direct visualization, magnification, and optimal lighting are just a few of the advantages over invasive surgical procedures. Other minimally invasive procedures, such as laser lithotripsy, urethral stenting, and basket retrieval of stones can be performed using the cystoscope.

EQUIPMENT AND INSTRUMENTATION

Flexible endoscopes (also called ultra-thin endoscopes) are used in male canine and feline cystoscopies. Cystoscopes made for the veterinary market measure 2.5 mm o.d. [7.5 French gauge (Fr)] and are 70–100 mm in length with a 1.2 mm instrument channel for 0.8 mm diameter accessories. This cystoscope will accommodate any dog that can be catheterized with an 8 Fr catheter. A lever is used for up/down movement of the distal tip for a broader viewing field, especially important for visualization in the bladder. The all-fiber-optic endoscopes also have light cable attachments at the control section, and the camera attaches via a C-clamp at the viewing lens. These ultra-thin endoscopes are now also available with video technology. This adaptable endoscope can also be utilized in smaller (less than 7 kg) dog and cat bronchoscopies. Although endoscopes are not recommended

Endoscopy for the Veterinary Technician, First Edition. Edited by Susan Cox.
© 2016 John Wiley & Sons, Inc. Published 2016 by John Wiley & Sons, Inc.

to be stored in their cases, the fragile nature of "ultra-thins" dictates that case storage may be the most secure location in a veterinary setting. Ensure that the endoscopes are completely dry (especially instrument channels) before storage.

Female dogs and cats require a rigid telescope for cystoscopy. Sizes can range from 2.8 mm (8.5 Fr) to 6.5 mm (19.5 Fr) o.d. with sheath. An intermediate size is 3.5 mm (10.5 Fr) with a length of 18 cm and a 1.2 mm (3.6 Fr) instrument channel. The 25° angle-of-view allows a wider area of the bladder to be examined in one field.

For endoscopic transcervical insemination in female dogs, a longer cystoscope is used. The working length is 29 cm and it has a 4 mm (12 Fr) o.d. with a 30° viewing angle. The sheath connects to a bridge that houses ports for fluid and biopsy instrumentation. A 6 or 8 Fr polypropylene urinary catheter fits in the instrument channel and is used for the insemination. If the endoscope requires lubrication before the procedure, make sure that it is non-spermicidal.

In order to visualize the urinary tract fully, especially the urethra, the cystoscope must have ports for infusion/removal of fluids, retrieval of uroliths or foreign bodies, and biopsy of masses or lesions. Flexible cystoscopes have a biopsy channel that is used for both flushing and retrieval. Keep in mind that the channel size of these endoscopes is small – biopsy forceps can be difficult to find and mechanical suction should not be used, as it could collapse the channel. Rigid cystoscopes for female dogs have a sheath that fits over the working length and attaches at the base. The sheath provides two ports for fluid infusion and retrieval and a biopsy/instrument channel.

Cystoscopy in felines is performed less frequently than in dogs because many lower urinary tract disorders in cats do not require the use of a cystoscope for correct diagnosis and management. Cystoscopy in cats is very similar to that in dogs but requires smaller endoscopes, such as an 8.5 Fr sheath and an 18 cm working length. Custom-made flexible endoscopes for male cats have a 1.1 mm (3.2 Fr) o.d. and a 55 cm working length. Be aware that some of these cystoscopes are not fully immersible for cleaning and disinfection. Check with the manufacturer if you are unsure.

Cystoscopy should be performed as a sterile procedure. Most rigid cystoscopes and light cables are autoclavable (check with the manufacturer). Flexible cystoscopes that are not autoclavable should go through high-level disinfection prior to the procedure and be placed on a sterile barrier drape. Sterile camera drapes are used over cameras and camera cords, or check with the manufacturer for camera sterilization guidelines. All participants handling the cystoscope require sterile gowns and gloves. Biopsy forceps, biopsy cassettes, guidewires, and other associated equipment should also be sterile.

Laser lithotripsy requires the use of a laser unit with laser fibers introduced through the endoscope's instrument channel. It is imperative that all personnel involved wear protective eye goggles and review safety training protocols before use. In addition to the endoscopy technician, an additional trained assistant must be assigned solely to the operation of the laser unit. The endoscopist and the laser assistant must be in constant communication while the laser is in use. A laser misfire too close to the endoscope could result in costly repairs.

Cystoscopes and accessories are delicate and costly – most manufacturers will not repair broken forceps. Port covers and catheter introducers come in small packages that can easily be lost. It is recommended to have dedicated carts or storage areas for cystoscopy equipment.

A 1 L bag of 0.9% saline in an ice–water bath should be available. In rare cases, excessive bleeding may occur, which leads to loss of visualization. Iced 0.9% saline instilled through the endoscope and into the bladder may aid in vasoconstriction.

A complete list of necessary supplies is in Box 8.1.

BOX 8.1 EQUIPMENT FOR UROGENITAL ENDOSCOPY

- Endoscopes
  - Male – flexible cystoscope
    - HLD prior to procedure; place on sterile drape
  - Female – rigid sterile 4152 telescope with sheath
- Component tower
  - Monitor on
  - Camera box or processor/light source
    - Patient info. entered
    - Ignition/light button depressed-light source
      - White balance
  - Image capture
    - Patient info. entered
- Sterile light cable
- Sterile camera or with camera drape (all-fiber-optic endoscopes)
- Large table with sterile table cover for instrumentation
- Sterile flexible biopsy forceps
- Sterile biopsy channel port cover
- Sterile fenestrated drape/cover drape
- Surgical gowns and surgical gloves
- 1 L 0.9% saline bags
  - Fluid line (female)
  - Fluid line with stopcock/syringe or pressure bag and extension set(s) (male)
- 0.9% saline in ice–water bath for infusion in case excessive bleeding occurs
- Clippers and chlorhexidine scrub and solution
- Dilute betadine/saline solution (male preputial flush)
- Sterile lubrication packets
- Sterile gauze
- Biopsy supplies
  - Sterile biopsy cassette
  - Container for uroliths
  - RTT/Culturette for sterile samples for culture

- Lithotripsy?
  - Laser unit
    - Assistant dedicated solely to laser unit support
  - Laser safety glasses – all personnel
  - Appropriate size laser fiber
  - Saline-soaked surgical towels to hold laser fiber on sterile field while not in use
- TCI?
  - 8 Fr polypropylene urinary catheter
  - Non-spermicidal lubrication
- Laboratory submittal forms
- Endoscopy report for recording observations

PATIENT PREPARATION

General anesthesia is required for all patients undergoing cystoscopy for patient comfort and equipment safety. Patients undergoing vaginoscopy should be evaluated for pain tolerance and can be heavily sedated or have general anesthesia. For transcervical catheterization for insemination (TCI), usually no sedation is needed. The patient is kept in a standing position with one or two assistants at tableside. These patients are usually in estrus and seem to accept the telescope with minimal discomfort.

If contrast radiography or fluoroscopy is planned, a radiograph should be performed on the morning of the procedure to check for fecal material in the colon. Warm water enemas should be given if feces is present. Patients should also be walked before anesthetic induction to observe the urine stream and to ensure an empty bladder for the start of the procedure.

ROOM PREPARATION

Cystoscopy in the female dog and male and female cat is performed with the endoscopist sitting at the end of the table. Patient positioning is dependent upon the endoscopist, either left or right lateral (as shown in Figure 8.1), or dorsoventral or ventrodorsal.

Male dogs are in either right or left lateral recumbency, with the endoscopist standing at tableside. The location of the video monitor will dictate the best position for the equipment tower and endoscopist. The assistant must also have room to retract the prepuce and administer fluids as the endoscope is advancing in the lower urinary tract.

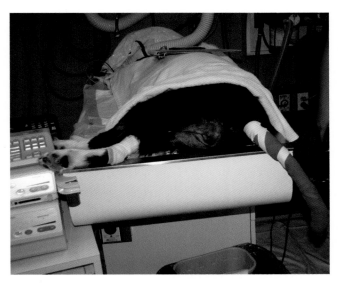

Figure 8.1 Female patient in right lateral recumbency in preparation for cystoscopy. The monitor is placed above and to the left of the table. The tail is wrapped and secured away from the area. The perineal area is carefully clipped, prepped, and placed as close to the end of the table as possible.

A 0.9% saline solution is constantly being infused or retrieved as the cystoscopy progresses. As a result, these procedures are best performed on a table with a grated surface. Absorbent pads placed on the floor will keep the area clean and accident-free.

The 1 L bags of 0.9% saline are hung on fluid poles and attached to ports on the endoscopes. For flexible cystoscopes (male dogs), a three-way stopcock is placed between an extension set and the main fluid line. A syringe is attached to the stopcock which the assistant fills with 0.9% saline from the bag and injects through the line as the cystoscope is advanced into the bladder. This allows the urethra to be fully distended, allowing for optimum visualization and safe passage of the cystoscope. Levers on the rigid cystoscope sheath allow the endoscopist to control fluid entry and exit. The assistant should pay close attention of the amount of fluid instilled and inform the endoscopist at 50–100 mL intervals, depending on the size of the patient. The bladder should also be palpated regularly so that over-distension does not occur. Air bubbles can also obscure visualization in the urinary tract and should be avoided. An alternative to the stopcock infusion method is to place a pressure infuser bag over the 0.9% saline bag.

If the endoscopist is delayed, the assistant can don sterile gloves and get the cystoscope ready for the procedure – attach the sheath, fluid line, camera drape, etc., and place on a sterile barrier drape away from excessive traffic.

PROCEDURE

- Anesthetized patient
- In correct position on table
- Carefully shave and prep the area, as shown in Figure 8.1
  - Clipper burn in these areas results in a longer recovery time
  - Cats and female dogs – perivulvar/testicular area
  - Male dogs – prepuce
    - Flush prepuce with dilute povidone–iodine or chlorhexidine solution
    - Secure dorsal pelvic limb away from field
- Fenestrated drape over field
  - Cover drape over patient may also be necessary to maintain sterility of equipment
- Endoscopist
  - Lead gowns under sterile gowns if fluoroscopy used
  - Laser protective goggles if laser used
  - Sterile gown and gloves, as shown in Figure 8.2

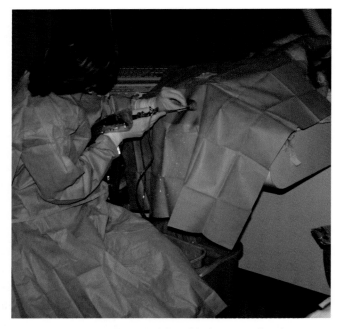

Figure 8.2 Endoscopist is seated at the end of the table for canine female cystoscopy. A fenestrated drape is placed over the endoscopy site, with the endoscopist wearing a sterile gown and gloves. A wastebasket is placed under the table to catch fluids as they drain from the telescope. A close-up of the telescope is shown in Figure 8.3.

- ○ Stance at table:
  - ▪ Female patient – end of table, sitting/standing
  - ▪ Male – side of table, monitor easily seen
- • Endoscope
  - ○ Sterile light cable, sterile camera, or camera drape, then camera attached to cystoscope, as shown in Figure 8.3
  - ○ 0.9% saline infusion
    - ▪ Flexible (male)
      - – Attach extension set to biopsy channel
        - ▫ Three-way stopcock at other end, then to fluid line for pressure infusion
        - ▫ Pressure infuser bag over liter saline
      - – Rigid (female)
        - ▫ Fluid line to port on sheath
        - ▫ Extension set to opposite port for fluid drainage
  - ○ Sterile gauze over tip for white balance
  - ○ Check focus and adjust if needed

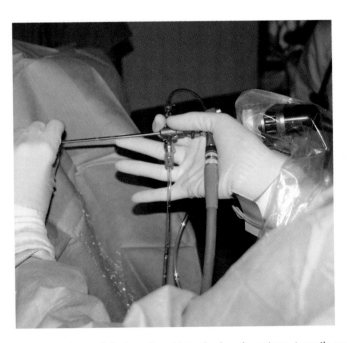

Figure 8.3 The telescope is carefully introduced into the female patient. A sterile camera drape is placed over the camera and camera cord with the fluid and drain lines attached to opposite ports on the telescope. Levers control saline infusion and outflow. A port cover is placed over the telescope's instrument channel and can also be opened/closed with a lever.

- ○ Sterile lubricant applied with gauze to distal tip/telescope
- ○ Biopsy port cover on biopsy channel port
- Vaginoscopy/cystoscopy – female
  - ○ Rigid cystoscope inserted dorsally, then aimed cranially and into the vaginal vault/vestibule
  - ○ Endoscopist digitally seals area around cystoscope for saline distension
  - ○ Standard appearance – vaginal vault
    - Pale pink mucosa
    - Distends readily with saline for optimum view
    - Hymenal remnant can bisect vaginal entrance
    - Urethral opening will be ventral to the vagina and appear as a longitudinal slit, as shown in Figure 8.4
  - ○ Observe for foreign bodies/mucoid material/ectopic ureters
  - ○ Standard appearance – urethra
    - Normal mucosa is light pink with vasculature easily seen
    - Mucosal folds should distend readily with fluids
  - ○ Trigone
    - Find ureteral openings

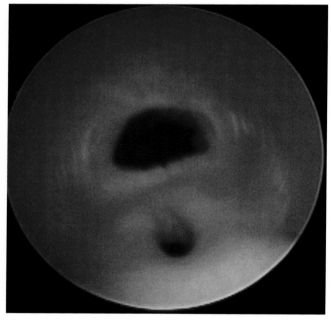

Figure 8.4 The vaginal vault houses the entrance to the vagina (the larger ovoid cavity), and the urethral opening, the smaller hole ventrally in the image. In some instances, the vaginal opening can be bisected by the hymenal remnant. Ectopic ureters can also be seen in this area, with urine "jetting" from the misplaced ureter.

- Located at dorsolateral aspect of the trigone area where the bladder mucosa begins and urethra ends, as shown in Figure 8.5
  - Easier to locate with fluid distension
  - Urine should be seen "jetting" from openings
- Bladder
- May need to drain urine and replace with 0.9% saline for visualization
- Standard appearance
  - Mucosa light pink with submucosal vessels apparent with fluid distension
- Cystoscopy – male dog
  - Assistant retracts prepuce
  - Cystoscope inserted into penis and luminal view achieved
    - Assistant infuses fluids to distend urethral lumen or pressure bag used
      - Keep track of amount instilled; inform endoscopist at predetermined intervals
  - Standard appearance – urethra
    - Light pink and uniform in shape throughout lumen
    - Slight narrowing at end of os penis and prostatic urethra
    - Distend readily and evenly with 0.9% saline infusion

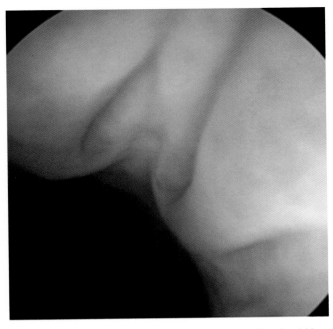

Figure 8.5 Right and left ureteral entrances seen at the trigone. Urine should be seen sporadically streaming from both ureters. Hematuria should be noted and classified as either unilateral or bilateral.

- ○ Trigone
  - ■ Find ureteral openings
    - – Located at dorsolateral aspect of the trigone area where the bladder mucosa begins and urethra ends, as shown in Figure 8.5
    - – Easier to locate with fluid distension
  - ■ Urine should be seen jetting from openings
- ○ Bladder
  - ■ May need to drain urine and replace with 0.9% saline for visualization
  - ■ Mucosa light pink with submucosal vessels apparent with fluid distension
- • Abnormal lower urinary tract findings
  - ○ Neoplasia
    - ■ Transitional cell carcinoma
      - – Commonly found at the trigone
      - – Can be obstructive
      - – Appears as a raised mass with fringe-like projections in the urethra, as shown in Figure 8.6
      - – Female dogs most commonly affected
      - – Urethral stents placed with fluoroscopic guidance can be palliative

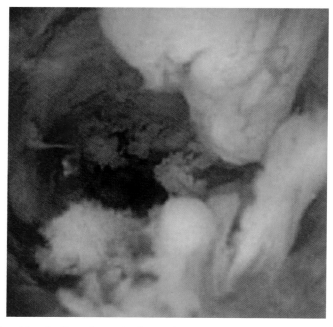

Figure 8.6 Transitional cell carcinoma in the urethra of a canine. This tumor can cause complete urethral obstruction with hematuria and straining noted by the owner. Urethral stenting utilizing interventional radiology can be palliative.

- Leiomyomas, adenocarcinomas and squamous cell carcinomas also seen
○ Inflammation
  - Urethritis and cystitis appear as hyperemic, thickened, and edematous mucosal walls
  - Petechiations, termed glomerulations, when observed in the bladder, may indicate an inflammatory process, as shown in Figure 8.7.
○ Prostatitis (male)
  - Appear as "roughened" and discolored mucosa at location of prostate
    – Can cause stricture and complete obstruction
○ Urethral and cystic calculi
  - Common in both dogs and cats
  - Varied sizes from gritty sand to large stones, as shown in Figure 8.8
  - Small stones removed with basket forceps
○ Uroliths/stone fragments
  - Basket retrieval forceps
    – Pass closed forceps just beyond stone, open forceps, retract slightly and enclose stone(s) into wire basket, as shown in Figure 8.9
    – Distend urethra with 0.9% saline infusion as endoscope is retracted

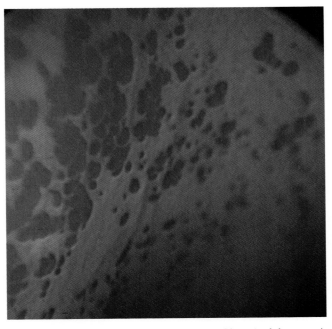

Figure 8.7 Inflammation of the bladder can be characterized by raised, hyperemic areas, also termed glomerulations. These areas are very friable and can cause loss of visualization in the bladder if grazed by the telescope.

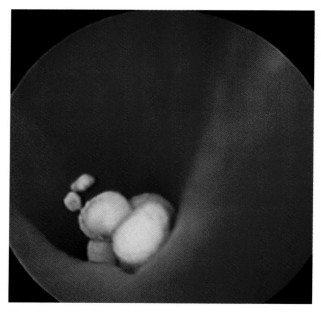

Figure 8.8 Uroliths of varying sizes seen in the urethra of a male dog. These stones can be extracted using a wire basket (see Figure 8.10) passed through the instrument channel of a flexible or rigid endoscope. The basket with stones is visualized as the endoscope is removed, ensuring a smooth extraction.

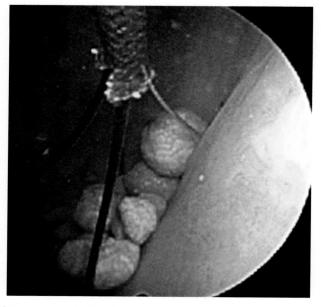

Figure 8.9 Basketing uroliths in the bladder. Depending on stone size, multiples may be gathered inside the basket and extracted. Fluid distension of the urethra as the basket/endoscope is being withdrawn is vitally important for the basket to pass smoothly.

- Cystoscope and forceps with stone removed as one unit
  - □ Never force or tug basket through urethra
- Collected into sterile RTT/container
- Removal of larger stones
  - Cystotomy
  - Laser lithotripsy
    - □ Laser fiber passed through the instrument channel
    - □ Stones fragmented and able to be basketed or voiding urohy-dropropulsion performed
- Ectopic ureter
  - Ureter enters at the urethra or in vagina (females) instead of trigone resulting in incontinence, as shown in Figure 8.10.
    - More females affected than males
    - More dogs than cats
    - May be unilateral or bilateral
    - Transection of ureter with endoscopic-guided laser to relocate to trigone area is minimally invasive and may be beneficial in selected patients
- Renal hematuria

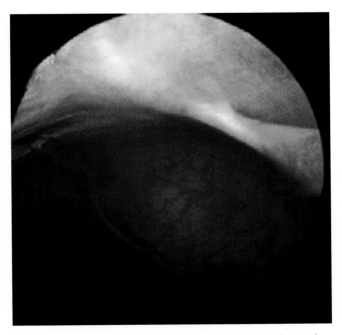

Figure 8.10 Ectopic ureter – ureteral opening tracks and empties into the urethra or has an abnormal configuration, resulting in incontinence. Ectopia can affect one or both ureters. Lasering of the affected ureter(s) can result in diminished incontinence.

- Blood seen coming through ureters from the kidneys
- Can be idiopathic
- Usually unilateral, but can be bilateral with blood seen coming from the ureters at different time points
  - Foreign body
    - Plant awns
    - Catheter remnant retrieval
      - Retrieval or basket forceps effective
- Biopsies, as shown in Figure 8.11
  - Check working order of forceps before use
  - Drain bladder to create folds
  - Biopsy samples will be small
    - Place samples on sterile biopsy cassettes, culture media, or RTT
    - Collected into sterile RTT/container
- Encourage endoscopist to complete endoscopy report

Transcervical Catheterization

- Patient standing with assistant gently supporting hind end
  - Owners can be present to assist and keep patient calm

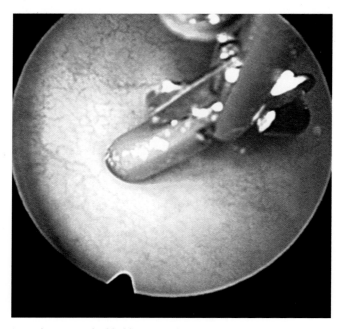

Figure 8.11 Biopsy forceps in the bladder. Note that the wings of the forceps are seen before the forceps are opened.

- 8 Fr polypropylene catheter placed in instrument channel
- Rigid telescope directed dorsally through vulva and into vagina
  - Vaginal lumen cavernous during estrus
- Follow dorsal median fold to cranial vagina/cervix
  - Appears as a rosette of mucosal folds at the cervical opening
  - Fluid accumulation may impede visualization
    - Aspirate or suction fluid for optimal view
    - Remove telescope and allow patient to sit and drain for several minutes
- Advance catheter into cervical opening, as shown in Figure 8.12
  - Position telescope parallel to cervical canal
  - Twisting motion may help advance catheter
  - Catheter should be advanced as far as possible without resistance
- Inject semen, then 1–2 mL of air to clear catheter
- Record ease of catheterization and instrumentation in endoscopy report

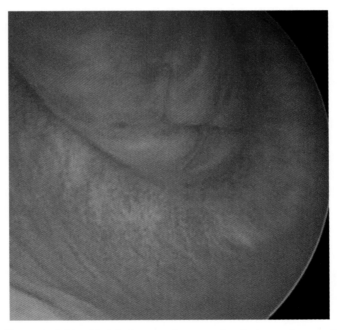

Figure 8.12 The cervix is identified during a vaginoscopy. A catheter can be passed into the rosette-shaped entrance during artificial insemination.

SAMPLE COLLECTION AND PROCESSING

Biopsy forceps and basket retrieval forceps used in cystoscopy are delicate owing to their small size and should be handled gently, especially when biopsying.

Forceps should pass through the instrument channel smoothly, and flexible cystoscopes should be in a neutral position while the biopsy forceps are in the channel. The cystoscope can then be flexed to the biopsy site when the forceps are out of the channel and the wings of the forceps are viewed. Excessive force on the up/down lever can stretch or break control wires, resulting in costly repairs. Always make sure that forceps and wire baskets are in working order before use.

Because of the size of the channel and biopsy forceps, tissue samples will be small. Placing samples in a tissue cassette will stabilize the sample. Samples for culture can be placed in a red-topped tube (RTT), or check with your reference laboratory for any other specifications.

Uroliths are placed in a small container such as an RTT with a tight lid.

POST-PROCEDURE PATIENT CARE

Patients with an obstructive neoplasia or inflammation from repeated cystoscope passes may benefit from placing a urinary catheter with a closed urinary system attached.

Clients should be informed that hematuria or frequent urination could occur for several days following the procedure.

COMPLICATIONS

Excessive hematuria despite repeated saline flushes can obscure the viewing field. Application of cold 0.9% saline flushes may be a benefit, or the procedure may have to be discontinued. Perforation of the urethra from inappropriate technique or neoplasia is rare. If necessary, a urinary catheter may be placed for 24-48 h or until the site heals.

SUGGESTED READING

Berent, A.C., Weisse, C., Mayhew, P.D., Todd, K., Wright, M., and Bagley, D. (2012) Evaluation of cystoscopic-guided laser ablation of intramural ectopic ureters in female dogs. *J. Am. Vet. Med. Assoc.,* **240**(**6**), 716–725.

Blackburn, A.L., Berent, A.C., Weisse, C.W., and Brown, D.C. (2013) Evaluation of outcome following urethral stent placement for the treatment of obstructive carcinoma of the urethra in dogs: 42 cases (2004–2008). *J. Am. Vet. Med. Assoc.,* **242**(**1**), 59–68.

Lulich, J.P., Adams, L.G., Grant, D., Albasan', H., and Osborne, C.A. (2009) Changing paradigms in the treatment of uroliths by lithotripsy. *Vet. Clin. North Am. Small Anim. Pract.,* **39**(**1**), 143–160.

Tams, T. and Rawlings, C.A. (2011) *Small Animal Endoscopy*, 3rd edn. Elsevier Mosby, St Louis, MO, pp. 507–561.

9   Laparoscopy and thoracoscopy

Katie Douthitt

William R. Pritchard Veterinary Medical Teaching Hospital, University of California-Davis, Davis,California, USA

The support provided by the veterinary technician, as part of the veterinary team, is integral to the success of any procedure. Familiarity with the procedure – indications and possible complications, timely set-up of equipment and supplies, anticipating common contingencies, knowing how to avoid malfunctions and resolving them when they occur – are all part of the technician's scope of responsibility. Endoscopic equipment is complex and has many points of possible malfunction, hence it is essential that the technicians involved in these procedures be adept at operating and troubleshooting every piece of equipment used.

LAPAROSCOPY

Definition of laparoscopy: a surgical procedure in which a fiber-optic instrument is inserted through the abdominal wall to view the organs in the abdomen or to permit a surgical procedure – from the Greek *lapara* meaning "flank or loin" and *skopein* meaning "to see" [1].

Laparoscopic-assisted surgery is a technique used typically for the examination, palpation, and biopsy of the abdominal organs and can be accomplished by partial exteriorization of the intestines through an enlargement of one of the abdominal port incisions or by placement of a laparoscopic wound retraction device [2, 3].

Endoscopy for the Veterinary Technician, First Edition. Edited by Susan Cox.
© 2016 John Wiley & Sons, Inc. Published 2016 by John Wiley & Sons, Inc.

Indications for Laparoscopy or Laparoscopic-Assisted Surgery [4–6]

The indications are similar to those for open abdominal surgery – laparotomy – and include:

- Visualization and examination of organs and gross disease processes
- Biopsy for histologic examination of organs such as liver (Figure 9.1), gallbladder, kidney (Figure 9.2), spleen, intestine (Figure 9.3), lymph nodes, pancreas and prostate
- Aspirates for cytologic examination of kidney, gall bladder, and lymph nodes

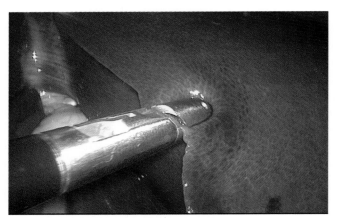

Figure 9.1 Liver biopsy with cup biopsy forceps.

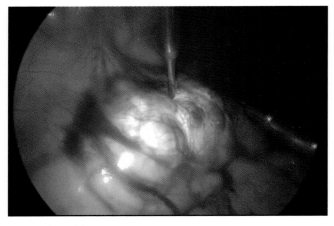

Figure 9.2 Laparoscopic orchiectomy.

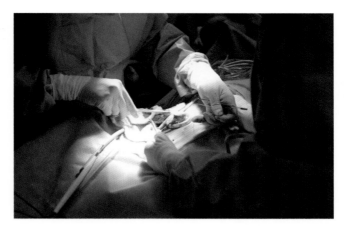

Figure 9.3 Laparoscopic kidney biopsy.

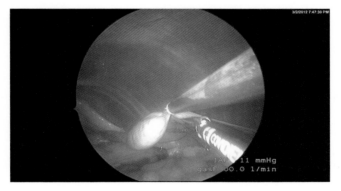

Figure 9.4 Laparoscopically assisted intestinal biopsy with wound retraction device.

- Biopsy and aspirate samples for culture
- Mass resection and biopsy
- Cancer staging
- Cryptorchid neuter and ovariectomy/ovariohysterectomy (Figure 9.4)
- Cystotomy/cystoscopy/cystopexy
- Adrenalectomy (Figure 9.5)
- Nephrectomy
- Cholecystectomy
- Gastrostomy tube placement
- Gastropexy
- Gastric foreign body removal
- Gastric dilatation and volvulus (GDV).

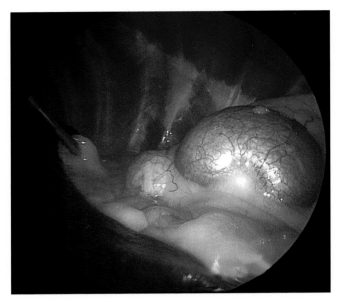

Figure 9.5 Laparoscopic adrenalectomy.

Contraindications for Laparoscopy (Absolute or Relative) [2,5,7a]

The contraindications for laparoscopy are essentially the same as those for any equivalent open surgical procedure. Some specific contraindications for laparoscopy include:

- Unmanageable hypercapnia
- Diaphragmatic or inguinal hernia
- Septic peritonitis
- Open abdominal wounds
- Prior abdominal surgery with multiple adhesions
- Large mass resections
- Patient size
- High body condition score – obesity
- Surgical team's level of skill
- Available equipment.

Advantages of Laparoscopy Over Laparotomy [5, 8, 9]

- Less invasive
- Less hemorrhage and trauma to tissues due to smaller incision sites
- Affords better visualization of the peritoneal cavity with pneumoperitoneum
- Is associated with less postoperative pain
- Less metabolic impairment

- Reduced postoperative morbidity
- Affords less opportunity for postoperative infection
- Lower incidence of wound dehiscence or hernia
- Shorter recovery time.

Disadvantages of Laparoscopy Over Laparotomy [5, 8, 9]

- Gas embolism
- Complications of pneumoperitoneum
- Increased length of procedures for novice practitioners
- Loss of tactile feedback when examining organs and tissues
- Less maneuverability of instruments
- Need for specialized equipment and associated expense
- Need for specialized training.

THORACOSCOPY

Definition of thoracoscopy: endoscopic examination of the chest cavity –f rom the Greek *thōrāx* (thoraco) meaning "chest" and *skopein* meaning "to see" [10].

Although the term thoracoscopy is often used to describe all procedures utilizing a scope to visualize the pleural cavity, efforts are being made by some in the medical community to separate or define more clearly the differences between the common terms thoracoscopy and video-assisted thoracic (thoracoscopic) surgery (VATS). For the purposes of this chapter, thoracoscopy will be used for medical diagnostic or therapeutic interventions and VATS will be used for minimally invasive thoracoscopic surgical procedures [11–13].

Indications for Thoracoscopy and VATS [13–23]

Indications for thoracoscopy and VATS are similar to those for the any open thoracic surgery – thoracotomy:

- Visualization and examination of organs and gross disease processes
- Diagnosis of pleural or pericardial effusion
- Aspirates for cytologic examination of effusions
- Biopsy for histologic examination of lymph nodes, pleura, lung, mediastinum
- Treatment of pyothorax
- Foreign body removal
- Resection of thoracic or anterior mediastinal masses
- Pericardiectomy (Figure 9.6), subphrenic, partial or full
- Thoracic duct ligation
- Lung biopsy, lobectomy, partial or full (Figure 9.7)
- Correction of pneumothorax
- Correction of persistent right aortic arch (PRAA)

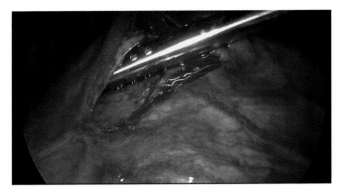

Figure 9.6 Thoracoscopic pericardiectomy, initial pericardial incision, and use of suction probe.

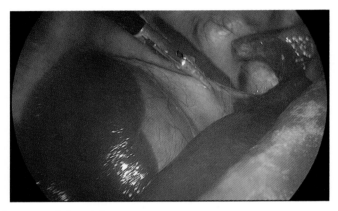

Figure 9.7 Thoracoscopic lung lobectomy.

- Ligation of patent ductus arteriosus (PDA)
- Pleurodesis.

Contraindications for Thoracoscopy and VATS [24, 25]

The contraindications for thoracoscopy are essentially the same as those for thoracotomy. Some specific contraindications for thoracoscopy include:

- Severe heart or pulmonary disease
- Patient unable to tolerate one-lung ventilation/unilateral collapse of the lung
- Pleural adhesions (also called pleurodesis, pleural symphysis, pleural sclerosis)
- Location of the lesion or disease process (central pulmonary lesions, involvement of the pericardium, diaphragm, or chest wall)
- Large lesions or masses
- Surgical team's level of skill
- Available equipment.

Advantages of Thoracoscopy/VATS Over Thoracotomy [5, 26–29]

- Less invasive
- Less trauma to tissues due to smaller incision sites
- Affords brighter, magnified visualization of the pleural cavity
- Associated with less postoperative pain
- Shorter recovery time
- Lower morbidity
- Affords less opportunity for postoperative infection and wound dehiscence
- Less incidence of postoperative lameness.

Disadvantages of Thoracoscopy/VATS Over Thoracotomy

- Increased length of procedures for novice practitioners
- Loss of tactile feedback when examining organs and tissues
- Less maneuverability of instruments
- Need for specialized equipment and associated expense
- Need for specialized training of surgeons and technical support staff.

LAPAROSCOPIC AND THORACOSCOPIC EQUIPMENT AND INSTRUMENTATION

The instrumentation and equipment used for endoscopic procedures are delicate and costly, hence all personnel involved in the use and maintenance of this equipment should be fully trained in the proper handling and care of each individual instrument (see Box 9.1) [7a,23,30–35].

> **BOX 9.1 INSTRUMENTATION AND EQUIPMENT USED FOR ENDOSCOPIC PROCEDURES**
> The instrumentation and equipment used for endoscopic procedures are delicate and costly, hence all personnel involved in the use and maintenance of this equipment should be fully trained in the proper handling and care of each individual instrument

The basic endoscopic equipment (listed in Box 9.2) required for laparoscopic or thoracoscopic procedures is the same as that for any endoscopic procedure; endoscope, camera, light source, viewing monitor, and documentation capability. A typical endoscopic tower is in Figure 9.8. Several companies manufacture endoscopic equipment, including Karl Storz, Richard Wolf, Olympus Surgical and Stryker.

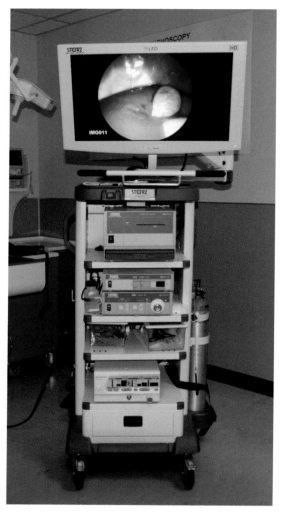

Figure 9.8 Endoscopic tower with an HD video and imaging system, including a medical-grade monitor, image capture unit, video processor, xenon light source, and gas insufflator.

BOX 9.2 MINIMUM EQUIPMENT REQUIRED FOR LAPAROSCOPIC AND THORACOSCOPIC EXAMINATION [2,32]

- Rigid endoscope
- Veress needle
- Cannula sleeves – threaded, smooth, or hybrid
- Trocars – pyramidal, conical, or blunt
- Light cable
- Light source

- Video camera/video processor/monitor
- Gas insufflator and tubing to deliver gas for pneumoperitoneum
- Compressed gas for pneumoperitoneum – laparoscopy only
- Documentation and archiving – a method for recording still images and/or videos of each procedure is not essential, but is highly recommended

Laparoscopes and Thoracoscopes

Endoscopes used for laparoscopy and thoracoscopy are typically rigid (as shown in Figure 9.9), although articulating hybrids are available; all come with a variety of outer diameters (o.d.), lengths, and angles of view.

Commonly used sizes in small animal practice:

- 3 mm o.d. × 14 cm – small dogs and cats
- 5 mm o.d. × 30 cm – most dogs and cats
- 10 mm o.d. × 30 cm – large and giant-breed dogs.

The most commonly used angles of view are 0 and 30°, as depicted in Figure 9.10; more obtuse angles of view are available.

Most rigid endoscopes come with standard rod and lens optics, although charge-coupled device (CCD) video and high-definition options are available. Many CCD video rigid endoscopes have an integrated single-cable camera and light source attachment, eliminating the need for a separate camera head and light cable.

Some rigid scopes have integrated working channels and offset eyepieces, termed operating laparoscopes. Many rigid endoscopes are available in auto-clavable and non-autoclavable models. Non-autoclavable endoscopes must be sterilized using cold sterilization such as glutaraldehyde (Cidex), accelerated hydrogen peroxide solution (Resert XL) ethylene oxide, or hydrogen peroxide gas plasma sterilization systems (Steris/Sterrad).

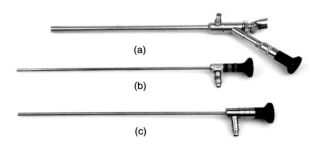

(a)

(b)

(c)

Figure 9.9 (a) Operating endoscope; (b) 30° endoscope; (c) 0° endoscope.

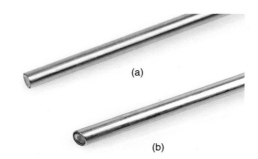

Figure 9.10 (a) 0° and (b) 30° endoscope angles of view.

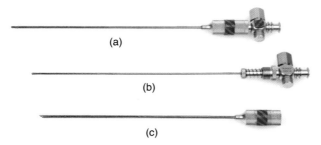

Figure 9.11 Veress needle: (a) assembled; (b) blunt stylet; (c) outer needle.

Veress Needle

The Veress needle shown in Figure 9.11 may be used to establish pneumoperi-toneum and pneumothorax. It consists of an outer needle with a sharp, beveled tip and a spring-loaded, retractable blunt stylet with a Luer attachment. After the needle has been introduced through the abdominal or thoracic wall and into the peritoneal or pleural cavity, the blunt stylet slides forward to protect inter-nal organs from inadvertent trauma. Proper function of the Veress needle should always be confirmed before each use and dull needles should be replaced.

Cannula Sleeves and Trocars [36, 37]

Cannulae and trocars are used for establishing and maintaining an access port into the peritoneal or pleural cavity.

As with many types of surgical equipment, cannulae and trocars come in a variety of options, including size, length, and type of material (metal or plastic), as shown in Figure 9.12. They can be reusable or disposable or even resposable (having a reusable cannula and disposable trocar). The sizes of the cannulae and trocars typically correspond to the size of the endoscope and the length used may depend on patient size, procedure to be performed, or simply surgeon preference. As risks associated with laparoscopy and thoracoscopy are largely considered to

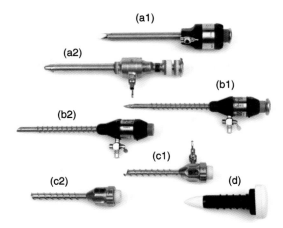

Figure 9.12 (a) Smooth cannulae with automatic one-way valves and Luer-lock insufflation attachments: (a.1) with a pyramidal tip trocar and (a.2) with a blunt tip trocar. (b) Hybrid threaded/smooth shaft cannulae with (b1) automatic one-way valves and (b2) Luer-lock insufflation attachments. (c) Threaded Storz Ternamian EndoTIP trocarless cannulae: (c.1) with automatic one-way valve and Luer-lock insufflation attachment and (c.2) without insufflation attachment. (d) Disposable threaded, valveless cannula (for thoracoscopy) with blunt trocar.

be highest during the initial establishment of pneumoperitoneum or pneumothorax, modifications of devices and techniques to insure a higher margin of safety are continually being explored. Box 9.3 provides a detailed list of types of cannulae and trocars.

BOX 9.3 TYPES OF CANNULAE AND TROCARS

- Cannulae:
  - Threaded
  - Smooth
  - Hybrid – threaded and smooth shaft combination
  - With or without an insufflation stopcock
  - Used without a trocar, e.g. Karl Storz Ternamian EndoTIP
  - Manual or automatic one-way valves
  - Silicone upper seal – no valve
- Trocars:
  - Cutting tips – shielded or unshielded
    - Pyramidal tip – sharp edges on three planes
    - Bladed tip – sharp edges on two planes
    - Sharp conical
  - Non-cutting tips:
    - Blunt tip
    - Blunt conical tip

Light Cables

Light cables facilitate the transfer of light from the main light source, e.g. halogen or xenon units, to the endoscope. Quality light cables are expensive and must be kept in good repair in order to achieve the maximum amount of light transfer. For types of light cables, see Box 9.4.

BOX 9.4 FIBER OPTIC AND FLUID-FILLED LIGHT CABLES

- Fiber-optic light cables use closely compacted non-coherent glass fibers to transmit light from the light source to the endoscope. Fiber-optic light cables are most commonly used in veterinary medicine. Many models are autoclavable
- Fluid-filled light cables use a liquid optical gel medium to transmit light. Although fluid-filled cables transmit about 30% more light, they conduct more heat, are non-autoclavable, more rigid, and fragile, and have a much higher purchase price [38]

Light cables, such as the example in Figure 9.13, come in a variety of lengths and diameters. Typical diameters range from 2 to 5 mm and lengths from 1.5 to 3 m.

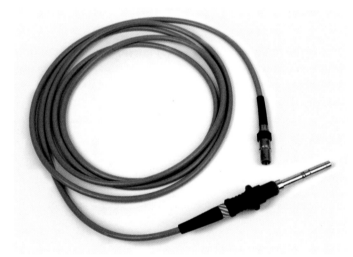

Figure 9.13 Fiber-optic light cable.

Light Source Units

Light source units generate high-intensity light, allowing good visualization during procedures. Two main types of light source units are used in veterinary endoscopic procedures: halogen and xenon (Box 9.5).

- *Halogen* – 150 W halogen light sources are good for the examination and diagnosis of gross disease processes in the peritoneal and pleural cavities. Halogen light sources produce more heat than their xenon counterparts.
- *Xenon* – A 100 or 300 W xenon light source provides a truer color representation of organs and tissues and are preferred for diagnostic or publication quality still images or video recordings. Although these light sources produce less heat than a halogen light source, special attention should always be given to the proximity of the tip of the endoscope to tissues and flammable surgical materials.

BOX 9.5 HALOGEN AND XENON LIGHT SOURCES

- *Halogen* – 150 W halogen light sources are good for the examination and diagnosis of gross disease processes in the peritoneal and pleural cavities. Halogen light sources produce more heat than their xenon counterparts.
- *Xenon* – A 100 or 300 W xenon light source provides a truer color representation of organs and tissues and are preferred for diagnostic or publication quality still images or video recordings. Although these light sources produce less heat than a halogen light source, special attention should always be given to the proximity of the tip of the endoscope to tissues and flammable surgical materials.

Typical settings and features of a light source unit include:
- Automatic and manual brightness controls
- Standby mode
- Lamp ignition control
- Lamp life meter
- Emergency lamp indicator – emergency lamp in use, no lamp warning, average lamp life
- Air pump – low, medium, and high settings (for use with gastroscopes)
- Water feed (for use with gastroscopes).

Video Cameras, Processors, and Monitors

In the early days of endoscopy, practitioners did not have the option of mounting a camera on an endoscope to facilitate viewing of the endoscopic image on a monitor: endoscopists had to look directly through the eyepiece. This limited viewing of the procedure to the endoscopist only and severely limited the ability to manipulate multiple instruments. Today, video cameras, processors and monitors are standard equipment.

Video camera systems (Box 9.6) are comprised of a camera control unit (CCU), camera head with connector cable (see Figure 9.14), endoscope adapter, and video monitor. Camera heads typically house one or three CCD chips.

BOX 9.6 VIDEO CAMERA SYSTEMS

- *Video camera*: Video camera systems are comprised of a camera control unit (CCU), camera head with connector cable, endoscope adapter, and video monitor. Camera heads typically house one or three CCD chips
- *Video processors*: Video processor systems are comprised of a video processor, camera head coupler, and endoscope adapters

---

Video processor systems are comprised of a video processor, camera head coupler, and endoscope adapters, as shown in Figure 9.15.

Typical settings and features of video cameras and processors:
- White balance control
- Automatic gain control
- Contrast setting
- Iris mode setting
- Image enhancement
- Image freeze
- Patient information input
- Still image capture
- Video display monitors.

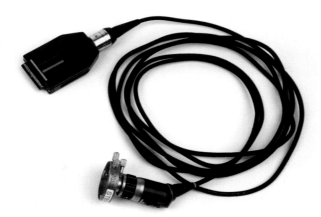

Figure 9.14 Three CCD chip camera head.

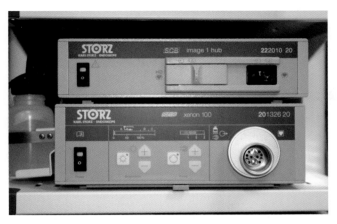

Figure 9.15 HD camera unit and 100 W xenon light source.

Video display monitors connect to the video camera or processor and are used to view the endoscopic procedure. Currently, monitors come in standard or high-resolution format and are available in a variety of sizes and styles. Preferences often depend on many factors, including compatibility with existing equipment and environments, image quality, size, price, and usage needs. Medical-grade monitors are highly recommended over consumer-grade monitors because specific design features make them optimal for the surgical environment and also compliance with government regulations and medical safety requirements. Medical-grade monitors generally have a sealed body with no vents or fans and smooth interfaces to impede trapping of particles, tissues, or fluids, allowing for better disinfection and maintenance of an aseptic surgical environment. They are typically made of more rugged materials than consumer monitors to reduce the possibility of damage while being manipulated in the surgical suite. Currently available monitor types are outlined in Box 9.7.

BOX 9.7 CURRENTLY AVAILABLE VIDEO DISPLAY MONITORS

- CRT – Cathode-ray tube
- LCD – Liquid crystal display
- OLED – Organic light-emitting diode
- Plasma – ionized gas cells
  - CRT monitors are still widely used, but are becoming less common. Although they may have excellent color reproduction, wide viewing angle, and no blurring or ghosting; they are overall much larger and heavier than their more compact counterparts.

- LCD monitors are becoming popular owing to their larger screen size, compact overall size and lower weight. LCD monitors, particularly HD (high-definition) models give very clear, crisp images with little or no screen flicker and can be mounted in a wider variety of locations than CRT monitors
- OLED monitors are a new medical display option. At -present only Sony has an OLED medical-grade monitor commercially available. The OLED technology can provide wider viewing angles, faster response time, less blurring of moving images, and truer color reproduction [9]
- Plasma displays are typically large, 32 in or greater. At present, plasma monitors are not utilized in operating room applications

Gas Insufflators and Tubing

Automatic gas insufflators (Figure 9.16) are used to establish and maintain pneumoperitoneum during laparoscopic procedures. They come with a variety of options, including various liter per minute (typically 20, 30, or 40 L/min), gas warming, smoke evacuation, and pressure release. Automatic insufflators monitor several parameters and can be set to accommodate patient size and possible considerations in health status. Common operating settings and monitors include the following:

- On/off
- Standby
- Maximum intra-abdominal pressure (set manually)
- Maximum gas flow rate (set manually)
- Gas supply level meter
- Total volume insufflated
- Tube obstruction alarm
- Excessive pressure alarm
- Low gas supply alarm.

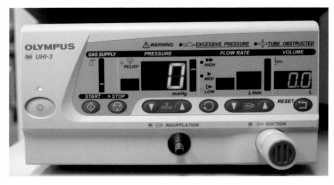

Figure 9.16 Gas insufflator.

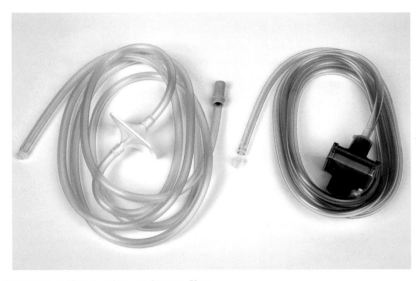

Figure 9.17 Insufflation tubing with microfilter.

Insufflation tubing (Figure 9.17) is single use and typically comes in 10 ft lengths; different models with a variety of connectors are available. Insufflation tubing should contain an integrated fluid barrier and bacterial/viral filter to avoid possible backflow of abdominal fluids and contaminants into the insufflator.

Insufflation Gases

Several gases may be appropriate for establishing and maintaining pneumoperitoneum [4, 9, 35]:

- Carbon dioxide (CO_2)
- Air
- Nitrous oxide
- Argon
- Helium.

CO_2 is the most commonly used gas in veterinary medicine, for several reasons [4, 9, 35]:

- High solubility
- Non-combustible
- Does not support combustion
- Natural metabolite
- Rapid removal from the body
- Lower risk of embolism.

Safety precautions with compressed gas cylinders are important (Box 9.8).

Documentation and Archiving

Documentation and archiving of procedures are an invaluable resource for reviewing cases, monitoring progress or resolution of disease, teaching, and sharing information with owners.

Documentation and archiving options are numerous and can be as simple as a DVD recorder attached to the video monitor output on the endoscopy tower, to advanced touchscreen input, HD, and PACS (picture archiving and communication system). Some method of documentation and archiving is highly recommended. See Figure 9.18.

Instrumentation

Laparoscopic and thoracoscopic procedures utilize specialized surgical instruments equivalent to the instrumentation used for laparotomy and thoracotomy

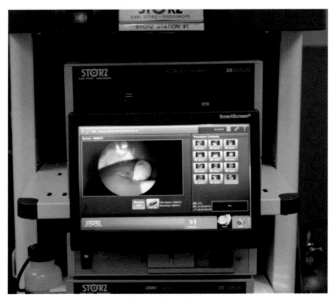

Figure 9.18 High-definition image capture with touchscreen.

procedures. These instruments come in a variety of sizes and lengths to coincide with the specific procedure, patient size, and cannula. Some instruments have rotation and locking mechanism options to enhance positioning and stability and are insulated for use with cautery. Many have modular handles and insertion tips enabling customization of instrumentation. They are easy to disassemble for cleaning and sterilization.

Specific instrumentation required will depend largely on the procedure being performed and surgeon preference. A list of basic instruments is itemized in Box 9.9. Figure 9.19 shows an example of an instrument tray, and Figures 9.20–9.24 demonstrate the variety of instruments available.

BOX 9.9 GENERAL LAPAROSCOPIC AND THORACOSCOPIC INSTRUMENTS AND SUPPLIES [3, 23, 25]

- Suction, suction/irrigation cannula
- Blunt palpation probe
- Cup biopsy forceps
- Punch biopsy forceps
- Dissection graspers
- Atraumatic graspers
- Retractor
- Right-angle forceps
- Babcock forceps
- Kelly forceps
- Metzenbaum scissors
- Hook scissors
- Needle holder
- Specimen retrieval bag
- Ligating loop
- Knot pusher
- Hemostasis supplies – direct pressure with blunt probe, gel–foam, suture, pre-tied suture loops, endoscopic clips or staples [4d]
- Core biopsy needle
- Electrocautery
- Electrosurgery unit, e.g. Ligasure
- Ultrasonic scalpel
- Suction/irrigation unit

Vessel Dissection and Sealing Devices[17, 32]

Ligating clips, endoscopic staplers, and bipolar tissue fusion devices are often used in minimally invasive surgical procedures. The ease of dissecting and ligating tissues compared with suturing in the pleural and peritoneal spaces makes these devices a favorable alternative. Examples of these devices are

- Gemini clip appliers (Microline Surgical)

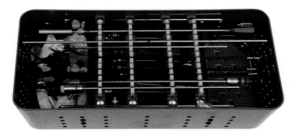

Figure 9.19 General laparoscopic instrument pack in autoclavable storage tray.

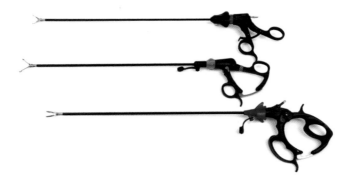

Figure 9.20 Surgical instruments for laparoscopy and VATS/thoracoscopy.

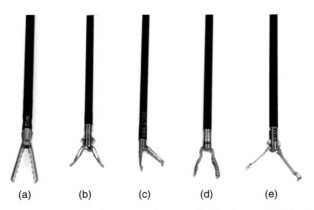

(a)   (b)   (c)   (d)   (e)

Figure 9.21 (a) Atraumatic wave side grasper; (b) curved Kelly forceps; (c) single-action grasping forceps; (d) fenestrated atraumatic graspers; (e) Babcock tissue forceps.

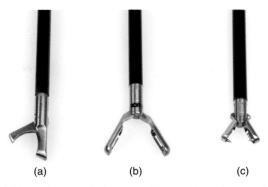

(a)   (b)   (c)

Figure 9.22 (a) Hook biopsy forceps; (b) fenestrated spoon biopsy forceps; (c) cup biopsy forceps with teeth.

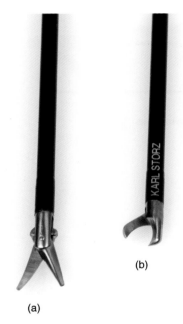

(b)

(a)

Figure 9.23 (a) Metzenbaum scissors; (b) hook scissors.

- EndoGIA endoscopic stapler (Covidien)
- LigaSure sealer (Covidien).

Each of these devices is available in different sizes and lengths. The size and length used is dependent on the size of the patient and the size and nature of the vessel or tissue being ligated or dissected. Examples are shown in Figures 9.25 and 9.26.

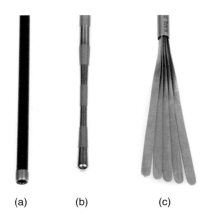

(a)   (b)   (c)

Figure 9.24 (a) Suction cannula; (b) blunt probe; (c) fan retractor.

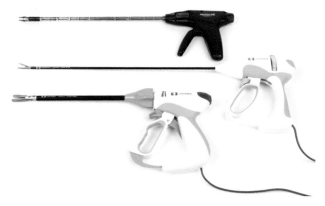

Figure 9.25 Ligating clip applier and vessel sealing devices.

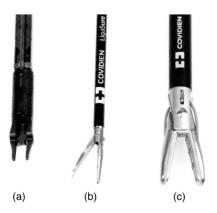

(a)   (b)   (c)

Figure 9.26 (a) Ligating clip; (b) dolphin tip vessel sealing device; (c) blunt tip vessel sealing device.

In the event that transition to an open procedure (laparotomy or thoraco-tomy) is required, laparotomy and thoracotomy instrumentation should be immediately available.

PATIENT PREPARATION

In general, patient preparations for a laparoscopic or thoracoscopic procedure are the same as those for any equivalent open surgery. Discussing the case with the surgeon well in advance of setup is ideal. This is the time to ask pertinent questions about the case, including any plans for additional procedures, order of multiple procedures, specific concerns or requirements for the patient, specific equipment needs, etc.

Prior to Anesthesia

- Allow the patient to void its bladder and bowels just prior to the procedure.
- Fasting of 8–12 h, depending on patient signalment and health status.
- Blood work, which may include a chemistry panel, complete blood count, and coagulation panel.
- Imaging diagnostics such as CT, MRI, X-ray or ultrasound.
- Anesthetic protocol established (see Chapter 3).

  owing to the inherent complications and physiologic effects of pneumoperi-toneum, pneumothorax, and one-lung ventilation (OLV), having an experienced anesthetist is essential.

Presurgical Patient Preparation [5, 32, 40]

Clip, scrub, and drape the patient to accommodate quick transition to an open procedure should it become necessary.

Clip and scrub for laparoscopy

Typically, a right lateral or ventral midline approach will be used for placement of the laparoscope. A ventral midline approach typically gives the best opportunity for visualization of the entire peritoneal cavity. A left lateral approach is less common owing to the location and possible traumatization of the spleen, but may be used for biopsy of the spleen and other left-sided organs such as left kidney and adrenal gland.

Clip and prepare the patient using a surgical aseptic technique.

For a ventral approach procedure, with the patient in dorsal recumbency, clip all of the fur at least 6 cm cranial to the xiphoid process down to the pubis and across and wide to the right and left lateral abdomen, as shown in Figure 9.27.

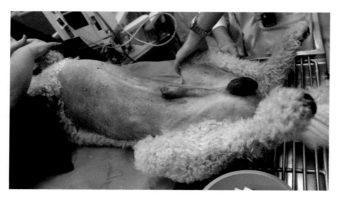

Figure 9.27 Clipping for ventral approach laparoscopic procedure.

For a right or left lateral approach, and with the patient in the appropriate right or left recumbency, clip all of the fur from dorsal to ventral midline starting about 6 cm cranial to the xiphoid process and down to the lateral pelvis.

Remove all loose fur. A Shop-Vac or hand-held vacuum is helpful. Be careful not to hold the vacuum nozzle too close to the patient's skin, as suctioning the skin can cause irritation or bruising.

Surgical scrub protocol

- Use gauze sponges soaked in antiseptic scrub and rinse solutions, perform an initial scrub to remove gross debris.
- Remember to flush the prepuce of male dogs with dilute antiseptic rinse, e.g. povidone–iodine or chlorhexidine solution diluted with sterile water or saline solution. Do not use alcohol as it is irritating to mucous membranes.
- Perform a final scrub of the entire surgical site using a standard surgical aseptic technique, making sure to allow the recommended contact time for the product used.

Clip and scrub for thoracoscopy/VATS [5, 26, 17, 32, 40]

- Depending on the procedure, a lateral intercostal or ventral transdiaphragmatic subxiphoid approach will be used for placement of the thoracoscope.
- Clip and prepare the patient using a surgical aseptic technique.
- For any thoracoscopic approach, ventral or lateral with the patient in dorsal recumbency, it is often a good idea to clip and scrub the entire ventral thorax and ventrum, from just above the thoracic inlet to the pubis and wide on each side to the dorsal midline. Having both hemispheres of the thorax clipped will

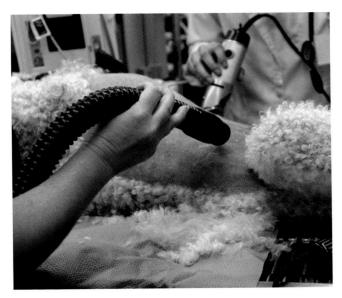

Figure 9.28 Vacuum hose position.

speed rescrubbing in the event of the need to access the opposite side for better access or if visualization is required.

- This wide shaving pattern (as shown in Figure 9.29) will insure easy rescrubbing in the OR in the event that an alternative thoracoscopic approach or transition to open thoracotomy is required.
- Remove all loose fur.
- Perform a surgical scrub protocol as in laparoscopy.

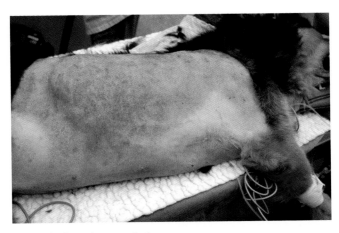

Figure 9.29 Clipping for lateral approach thoracoscopy.

PATIENT POSITIONING

After the patient has been clipped and scrubbed, it can be moved into the operating room and positioned on the surgery table as shown in Figures 9.30 and 9.31. When electrosurgical devices requiring a grounding plate are to be used, be sure that the grounding plate is in place prior to placing the patient on the operating table and that there is good contact with the patient once it has been positioned. Depending on the procedure, the patient may need to be repositioned. When using a tilting operating table, the patient should be firmly secured to the table by more than the typical leg ties used for many surgical procedures. Restraints such as molded patient positioners, padded Velcro straps or 2 in white tape with surgery towels as padding can be used. Straps should be kept clear of the surgical field and not interfere with expansion of the lungs and ventilation, with placement low across the pelvis and high on the shoulders.

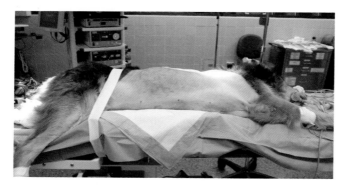

Figure 9.30 Patient position for right lateral approach thoracoscopy.

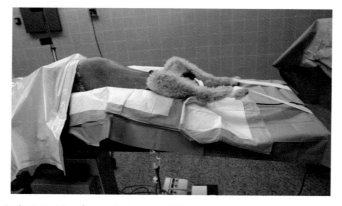

Figure 9.31 Patient position for ventral approach laparoscopy.

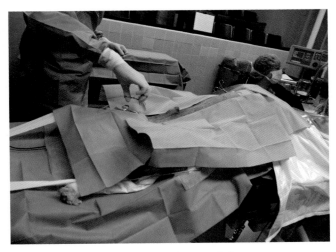

Figure 9.32 Example of initial draping for ventral approach laparoscopy.

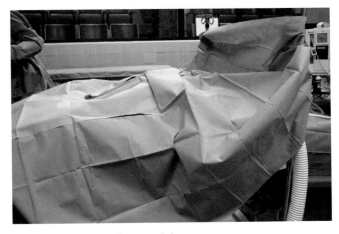

Figure 9.33 Final draping for ventral approach laparoscopy.

A final surgical scrub should be performed just prior to draping the patient. An example of draping for laparoscopy is shown in Figures 9.32 and 9.33.

LAPAROSCOPY PROCEDURE

Considerations During Laparoscopy [25, 36, 37, 41–43]

One of the main differences and considerations during laparoscopy compared with open laparotomy is the effects of pneumoperitoneum, most commonly hypercapnia due to increased absorption of CO_2 and a decreased tidal volume due to pressure on the diaphragm. Other complications are associated with perforation of an organ or venous structure or are consequences of prolonged excessive intra-abdominal pressure, and include:

- Subcutaneous empyema
- Insufflation of intestines
- Perforation of bowel
  - Peritonitis
  - Septicemia
- Perforation of vessels, e.g. mesenteric and iliac vessels, aorta, inferior vena cava
  - Gas embolism
  - Hemorrhage
- Perforation of spleen
  - Gas embolism
  - Hemorrhage
- Perforation of diaphragm
  - Herniation
  - Pneumothorax
- Reduced venous return with resultant ischemia and hypoxia
- Vasovagal response
- Port site metastasis.

Abdominal Access and Creation of Pneumoperitoneum [9, 25, 36, 41, 44]

For a right lateral approach, proper mid-abdominal placement of the Veress needle or cannula and trocar will typically be determined using the costal arch of the ribs with location of the lateral pelvis and ventral abdomen as anatomic landmarks. For a ventral approach, entrance at the caudal umbilicus is sometimes favored.

Creation of the pneumoperitoneum and insertion of trocars are widely considered the most critical point in the laparoscopic procedure; it is at this time that most injuries to organs and vessels occur. An internal view of placement is shown in Figures 9.34 and 9.35.

Initial pneumoperitoneum can be accomplished using a variety of methods: use of a Veress needle (blind technique), insertion of a blunt trocar and cannula via cut down, known as the "open" or Hasson technique, and techniques that utilize a cannula without the use of a trocar, e.g. the Ternamian cannula. There is much debate regarding which method is safer, and so far the decision is mainly dependent on surgeon comfort and experience with a particular technique.

Veress Needle Techniques

Confirmation of proper Veress needle placement in the peritoneal cavity can be established by a variety of methods. These methods are often used in tandem

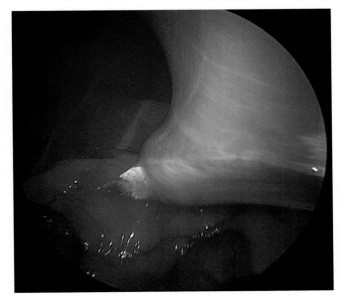

Figure 9.34 Introduction of trocar and cannula under direct visualization.

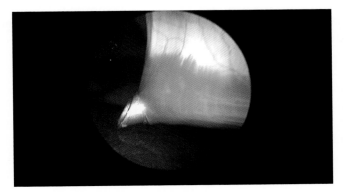

Figure 9.35 Introduction of trocar and cannula under direct visualization.

with each other, thus providing the surgeon with several "checks" to insure proper placement of the needle:

- The hanging drop technique – Flush the needle with sterile saline, then place a drop of sterile saline on the hub of the Veress needle. When the needle has penetrated the abdominal wall, the negative pressure of the peritoneal cavity will pull the drop into the cavity.
- The aspiration test – A syringe filled with a small amount of sterile saline is attached to the Veress needle. If placement is correct, injection of saline into the peritoneal space should meet with little resistance and nothing should be

returned upon aspiration. If saline is returned, the needle may be situated in a pocket in the abdominal wall and repositioning of the needle is required. If bowel contents, urine, or blood are aspirated, conversion to laparotomy may be required.

- "Click" method – While advancing the Veress needle through the abdominal wall, the surgeon listens for the "click" of the spring-loaded stylet coming out of the needle sheath as it meets with less resistance passing through the various muscle walls.
- Intra-abdominal pressure reading – Confirmation of correct placement of the Veress needle can be established by attaching the CO_2 supply to the Luer lock of the needle and monitoring the abdominal pressure reading on the insufflator. If the Veress needle is correctly placed in the peritoneal cavity, the pressure reading should be low (<5 mmHg). If the pressure reading is above 5 mmHg, the needle may be situated in the abdominal wall or hollow viscus.

Open or Hasson Technique

The open or Hasson technique has gained popularity due to the surgeon's ability to confirm visually entry into the peritoneal cavity and use of blunt, in place of sharp, trocars to establish an access port and pneumoperitoneum.

Modified Hasson techniques typically involve a combination of small incisions, blunt dissection and introduction of a cannula with a blunt-tipped trocar or trocarless cannula (Ternamian cannula) into the peritoneal cavity.

The CO_2 supply is attached directly to the cannula and pneumoperitoneum is established. These techniques avoid blind introduction of sharp instruments into the peritoneal cavity.

Prior to abdominal insufflation, the insufflator settings and unit functionality should be checked. The maximum insufflation pressure is typically set to 10–12 mmHg and should be set no higher than 15 mmHg at a flow rate of approximately 1–3 L/min.

Once pneumoperitoneum has been established and the laparoscope has been advanced into the abdominal cavity, placement of the remaining cannulae can proceed under direct visualization with the laparoscope, as shown in Figure 9.36.

THORACOSCOPY/VATS

Considerations During Thoracoscopy/VATS

Possible complications from thoracoscopy/VATS include the following [35]:
- Infection
  - Port insertion sites
  - Empyema

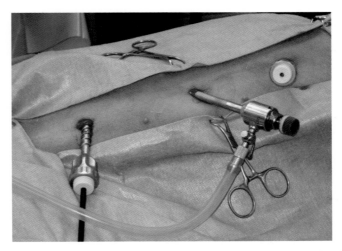

Figure 9.36 Port placement for laparoscopic ovariohysterectomy. The patient's head is toward the right of the image.

- Trauma
  - Nerve injury
    - Intercostal
    - Phrenic
  - Organs and vessels
    - Heart
    - Lungs
    - Esophagus
    - Trachea
    - Pulmonary, intercostal pleural vessels
- Hemorrhage
  - Intercostal vessels, pleural vessels, biopsy site
  - Pulmonary vessels, lung lobe
  - Pericardium, heart, PDA
  - Neoplasia
- Air leak
- Pneumonia
- Atelectasis

Thoracic Access and Creation of Pneumothorax [5, 17, 32]

Creation of pneumothorax can be achieved by use of a Veress needle with the stopcock valve open or by using a thoracoscopic valveless cannula. Either is placed in the thoracic cavity, allowing air to be introduced passively or by insufflation into the pleural space. The Veress needle technique is associated with

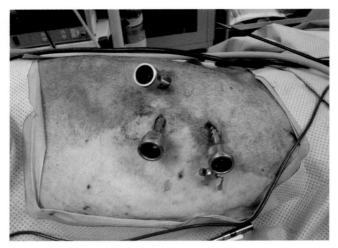

Figure 9.37 Thoracoscopic intercostal port placement for lateral approach.

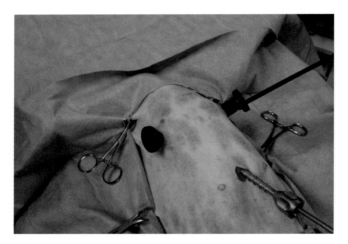

Figure 9.38 Subxiphoid and intercostal port placement for ventral approach.

greater risk of pulmonary trauma. Two examples of portal placement are shown in Figures 9.37 and 9.38.

One-Lung Ventilation (OLV) [45]

The ability to provide OLV may be necessary to increase visualization during thoracoscopic procedures (see Chapter 3 for more information).

The same endoscopic equipment – camera, camera head, and light source – can be utilized for the bronchoscopic placement of the OLV device. If you have two camera heads or are using a video bronchoscope or thoracoscope, maintaining the sterility of the camera head will not become an issue as it will not be used for both endoscopes. If you need to use the same camera head for the bronchoscope and thoracoscope, careful handling is essential to maintain the sterility of the camera head and cable. A sterile sleeve or drape may be used to cover the camera head and cable to protect them from contamination during the bronchoscopic placement of the OLV device and then carefully removed before attaching the camera to the sterile thoracoscope. Another option when only one camera head is available is to sterilize the bronchoscope (by whatever available method the scope is rated for – glutaraldehyde, ethylene oxide, Sterrad, steam), and lay it on a sterile drape. Be sure the bronchoscopist is wearing sterile gloves when handling the scope to avoid contamination of the camera head.

Equipment Preparation

Each piece of endoscopic equipment often has several features and options for operation. It is important that the technical team be familiar with the settings and options of each piece of equipment. Read the owner's manuals, operate the equipment, and explore the settings and features well in advance of a procedure. It is difficult and frustrating to troubleshoot malfunctions during a procedure if you are unfamiliar with how the equipment functions.

Ideally, two to three technicians should be available to assist with laparoscopic and thoracoscopic procedures – a technician to act as anesthetist, a technician to run the endoscopic and ancillary equipment, and a technician to scrub into the procedure if needed.

All instruments and equipment should be collected and available prior to the procedure. A good practice is to have, when possible, duplicate instruments and supplies ready to use in case of malfunction, breakage, or misplacement outside of the sterile field.

It is often difficult to test the functionality of sterile endoscopic instruments just prior to a procedure. Regular maintenance and testing of instruments at clean-up and before sterile reprocessing are good practice.

Perhaps one of the most common issues with any endoscopic equipment is the disconnection or incorrect connection of cables and wires to their appropriate units. The camera, monitor, and documentation system, for example, must all be properly connected to each other so that information from the endoscope can be transferred via the camera to the monitor and captured by the documentation system.

Cameras, monitors and documentation systems have several connection options: S-Video, RGB, DVI, HDMI, etc. Having a cable management system such as colored zip ties or Velcro straps to keep cables from coming loose or becoming entangled and difficult to trace along with a schematic of proper connections are helpful.

Typically, connections will go from the camera to the documentation system to the video monitor. In case the documentation unit fails, it is a good idea to have a direct connection between the camera and the video monitor, one that is independent of the documentation system, so that visualization of the procedure can continue without needing to wait for the problem with the image capture unit to be resolved.

Tower positioning

To facilitate ease of viewing, positioning of the endoscopic tower should typically be on the opposite side of the patient to the surgeon, so that the surgeon is facing the video monitor, as shown in Figure 9.39. Whenever possible, connect the tower to outlets that will permit repositioning of the tower if necessary without the need to unplug and reconnect the equipment, for example, multiple procedures requiring different angles of view. Make sure that cables are not an impediment to the movement of the surgeon/surgical team or ancillary equipment and are not stretched tight or easily pulled out of their sockets and connections.

Equipment Assembly

Once the patient is positioned and draped and the correct position of the endoscopy tower has been established, the instrument table drapes and all necessary surgical and endoscopic equipment can be opened, assembled, and tested for functionality. These steps should include:

- Confirmation that the correct patient information has been entered into the documentation unit.
- Confirmation that the camera is working and properly connected to the video monitor and imaging system.

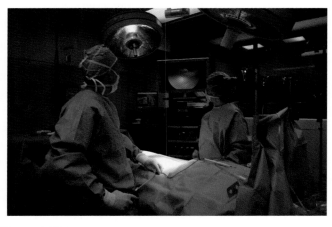

Figure 9.39 Tower position.

- Connection of the camera head and light cable to the endoscope.
  - Using a sterile technique, the camera head is attached to the endoscope eyepiece and should be positioned so that the top of the camera head is kept upright. This position allows for proper orientation when viewing the peritoneal and pleural cavities.
- The light cable should be securely attached to the endoscope light post.
- Connection of the camera and light cable to the main units on the tower.
  - While maintaining the sterile field, the distal connectors of the light cable and camera head are handed off to be connected to the camera control unit and light source on the tower.

Once the camera and light cable have been connected to the main units on the tower:

- Power on the camera control unit and light source.
- Verify that there is a live video feed from the endoscope to the video monitor.
- Ignite the lamp by depressing the lamp/ignition button on the light source unit.
- White balance the camera – perform this step with the endoscope held in front of a white object, e.g. a sterile gauze sponge.
  - Some camera systems have a white balance button located on the central control unit, others have white balance controls located on the camera head.
- Focus the image at the camera head.
- Check that the position of the image is centered on the monitor.
- Recheck proper equipment functionality and settings, such as insufflator, LigaSure or cautery units.

Common Equipment Considerations During the Procedure

Securing light cables, camera head cord, suction tubing, and other equipment to the sterile field

Light cables, camera head cords, suction tubing, and other equipment that is attached to units outside of the sterile field need to be secured so that they do not slide off of the table and fall to the floor or become unsterile. Some patient drapes have built-in loops through which cables and tubing can be threaded. Another option is to wrap the cables snugly in part of the sterile drape or with any soft, sterilized material such as vet wrap or a 4 × 4 gauze sponge and securing them by clamping the vet wrap/gauze to the patient drape with towel clamps or hemostats. An example is shown in Figure 9.40.

Lens fogging [46]

Owing to temperature and humidity variations, fogging of the lens can occur on insertion of the endoscope into the peritoneal or pleural cavity. Fogging typically resolves after a few minutes, when the endoscope acclimates to the patient's

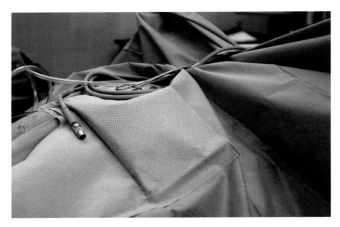

Figure 9.40 Cables and tubing secured with hemostats and sterile drape.

body temperature; fogging can, however, prolong procedures and diminish the surgeon's ability to perform examination and diagnostics.

During some procedures, simply bumping the lens of the endoscope gently against tissue, such as omentum, will clean the lens and renew visibility. Alternatively, there are many commercially available options, e.g.:

- Commercial scope warmers
- Anti-fogging solutions
- CO_2 humidification and warming
- Warm saline baths.

Light transmission

Although the automatic setting on the light source unit will often compensate acceptably, adjustments to the level of light transmission may need to be made during a procedure. This may be due to variations in the size of different regions of the peritoneal or pleural cavity, variation of equipment, surgeon preference, or distance needed from the endoscope to the area of focus. If light transmission is low:

- Check that the light source is powered on and the lamp has been ignited.
- Check that the light source is not in "standby" mode.
- Check the light cable connections at the scope and the light source.
- Check that the endoscope or light cable is transmitting light appropriately. This can be done by attaching an alternative light cable to the endoscope and light source unit and reassessing light transmission and/or attaching an alternative endoscope to the light cable and camera head.

Blurred image

A blurred image may be due to several factors:

- Camera head has not been focused.

- The tip of the endoscope has debris, blood, or other tissue obscuring the lens.
- Debris is present on the eyepiece or camera head.
- Damage to the lenses of the endoscope or camera head.

Off-center image or loose camera head to endoscope connection
If the image is not centered on the monitor screen, or there is movement between the endoscope and camera head, check that the camera head and endoscope are correctly connected and that the camera head is well seated on the eyepiece. Recheck and adjust the camera head position, making sure that the top of the camera head is in an upright position to insure proper orientation of view during the procedure.

Insufflator
The automatic insufflator will give an alarm when the intra-abdominal pressure readings exceed maximum settings. Possible causes of overpressure readings may include the following:
- Kinking or occlusion in the insufflation tubing.
- Veress needle or cannula Luer lock valve is in the off position.
- Veress needle or cannula has been backed out of the peritoneal cavity and into the intra-abdominal tissue.
- The technician should routinely check the insufflator readings and not depend solely on alarms to alert them to problems. Not being aware and setting the maximum intra-abdominal pressure on the insufflator too high will not result in an alarm sounding, but can cause serious injury or death to the patient.
- Low gas supply alarm.
- The technician should be aware of gas supply in the (CO_2) tank prior to the procedure. A back-up tank should always be available.

SAMPLE COLLECTION AND PROCESSING

The technician often works in tandem with the surgeon to acquire and prepare samples during the procedure. Improper collection, handling, and preparation of biological specimens can severely undermine the overall success of a procedure and the ability of the veterinarian to make a definitive diagnosis and treatment plan for the patient. Therefore, it is important that the technician be aware of correct handling and processing of samples.

Some general considerations for specimen handling are as follows:
- Careful handling of delicate tissues should be employed to avoid crush artifact.
- Samples should be placed in the appropriate preservative and container as soon after acquisition as possible, e.g. biopsy cassette, 10% formalin, isotonic NaCl, culture medium.

- Laboratories may differ in their requirements for submitting samples – be aware of these requirements prior to preparing specimens for submission.
- The distance from the operating room to the laboratory will make a difference to how a sample is initially preserved and transported.
- Laboratory submission forms should be completely filled out, as clinical information and tests requested are essential to an accurate reading and laboratory diagnosis.

POSTPROCEDURE EQUIPMENT CARE

Documentation on the procedure should be archived or uploaded to the patient record or other storage medium.

All equipment on the endoscopic tower should be wiped down and disinfected; be sure to include the shelves and surfaces of the tower itself.

All endoscopes and surgical equipment should be carefully disassembled (as shown in Figure 9.41) and cleaned. Be sure to disassemble trocars, Veress needles and modular surgical instruments fully before cleaning and sterilization.

POSTOPERATIVE PATIENT CARE [5,8,19]

Some of the most desirable aspects of minimally invasive endoscopic procedures over open surgery are an overall reduction in postoperative pain, lower morbidity, reduction of complications, and a shorter postsurgical recovery period.

With that said, patients should still receive postoperative analgesics and be monitored for postoperative complications as if they had undergone laparotomy or thoracotomy, including:

- Risks associated with general anesthesia
- Dehiscence of sutures

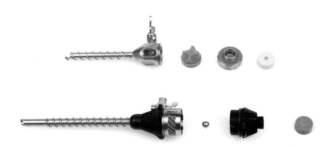

Figure 9.41 Disassembled cannula.

* Herniation
* Hemorrhage due to iatrogenic trauma or failure of hemostatic interventions
* Surgical wound infection
* Subcutaneous empyema
* Thoracic air leak
* Chest tube complications.

REFERENCES

1. Laparoscopy. *Oxford Dictionaries*, www.OxfordDictionaries.com, accessed April 2010.
2. Gower, S. and Mayhew, P. (2008) Canine laparoscopic and laparoscopic-assisted ovariohysterectomy and ovariectomy. *Compend. Contin. Educ. Vet.*, **30(8)**, 430–432.
3. Gower, S.B. and Mayhew, P.D. (2011) A wound retraction device for laparoscopic-assisted intestinal surgery in dogs and cats. *Vet. Surg.*, **40(4)**, 485–488.
4. Mayhew, P. (2009) Surgical views – laparoscopic and laparoscopic-assisted cryptorchidectomy in dogs and cats. *Compend. Contin. Educ. Vet.*, **31(6)**, 274–281.
5. Teoh, B., Sen, R., and Abbott, J. (2005). An evaluation of four tests used to ascertain Veres needle placement at closed laparoscopy. *J. Minim. Invasive Gynecol.*, **12(2)**, 153–158.
6. Vilos, G.A., Ternamian, A., Dempster, J., and Laberge, P.Y.; The Society of Obstetricians and Gynaecologists of Canada (2007) Laparoscopic entry: a review of techniques, technologies, and complications. *J. Obstet. Gynaecol. Can.*, **29(5)**, 433–465.
7. SAGES Surgical Wiki, www.sageswiki.org. (a) *Guidelines for Diagnostic Laparoscopy* (2011), accessed 8 October 2012; (b) *Laparoscopy Troubleshooting Guide*, Society of American Gastrointestinal Endoscopic Surgeons, Developed and Distributed by the SAGES Continuing Education Committee, accessed 8 October 2012; (c) *Practice/Clinical Guidelines: Guidelines for Diagnostic Laparoscopy*, Society of American Gastrointestinal and Endoscopic Surgeons (SAGES) (2007), accessed 10 October 2012; (d) *Principles of Laparoscopic Hemostasis*, accessed 10 October 2012.
8. Basilio, P. (2009) Minimally invasive, minimal drawbacks. *Vet. Forum*, **26(11)**, 8–14.
9. Mayhew, P. (2008) Modified sutureless Hasson technique for abdominal access. *Compend. Contin. Educ. Vet.*, **30(8)**.
10. Merck (2013) *Thoracoscopy and Video-Assisted Thoracoscopic Surgery*, www.merckmanuals.com, accessed 2 April 2013.
11. Lewis, R.J. (1996) VATS is not thoracoscopy. *Ann. Thorac. Surg.*, **62(2)**, 631–632.
12. Malhotra, R. (2011) *Medical Thoracoscopy*, http://emedicine.medscape.com, accessed 2 April 2013.
13. Twedt, D. (2001) *Gastrointestinal Endoscopy in Dogs and Cats*. Ralston Purina, St Louis, MO.
14. Dieter, R.A. Jr and Kuzyçz, G.B. (1997) Complications and contraindications of thoracoscopy. *Int. Surg.*, **82(3)**, 232–239.
15. Garcia, A. and Mutter, D. (2003) *Video Monitor*. WeBSurg.com, www.websurg.com/doi-ot02en307a.htm, accessed 7 October 2012.
16. Moore, A.H. and Ragni, R.A. (eds) (2012) *Clinical Manual of Small Animal Endosurgery*. Blackwell Publishing, Oxford.
17. Mayhew, P., Dunn, M., and Berent, A. (2013) Surgical views: thoracoscopy: common techniques in small animals. *Compend. Contin. Educ. Vet.*, **35(2)**, E1.

18. Mayhew, P.D., Culp, W.T., Mayhew, K.N., and Morgan, O.D. (2012) Minimally invasive treatment of idiopathic chylothorax in dogs by thoracoscopic thoracic duct ligation and subphrenic pericardiectomy: 6 cases (2007–2010). *J. Am. Vet. Med. Assoc.*, **241**(7), 904–909.

19. McCarthy, T.C. (ed.) (2005) *Veterinary Endoscopy for the Small Animal Practitioner*. Elsevier Saunders, St Louis, MO.

20. Monnet, E. (2009) Interventional thoracoscopy in small animals. *Vet. Clin. North Am. Small Anim. Pract.*, **39**(5), 965–975.

21. Pizzi, R. (2009) *Laparoscopic Correction of a Canine Gastric Dilatation and Volvulus (GDV)*. Veterinary Laparoscopy, www.veterinarylaparoscopy.com, accessed 12 October 2012.

22. Sony Corporation of America (2015). *Product Catalog*. www.sony.com, accessed 17 April 2015.

23. Stryker (2015) Endoscopy. *Product Catalog*. www.stryker.com, accessed 17 April 2015.

24. Abarkar, M., Sharifi, D., Kariman, A.A., et al. (2007) Evaluation of intraoperative complications in pericardiectomy with transdiaphragmatic thoracoscopic approach in dog. *Iran. J. Vet. Surg. (IJVS)*, **2**(4), 62–68.

25. Lansdowne, J.L., Mehler, S.J., and Bouré, L.P. (2012) Minimally invasive abdominal and thoracic surgery: principles and instrumentation. *Compend. Contin. Educ. Vet.*, **34**(5), E1.

26. Bennett, A. (2009) Minimally invasive surgery – laparoscopy and thoracoscopy. In *Proceedings of the SEVC Southern European Veterinary Conference*, 2–4 October 2009, Barcelona.

27. De Rycke, L.M., Gielen, I.M., Polis, I., Van Ryssen, B., van Bree, H.J., and Simoens, P.J. (2001) Thoracoscopic anatomy of dogs positioned in lateral recumbency. *J. Am. Anim. Hosp. Assoc.*, **37**(6), 543–548.

28. Richard Wolf Medical Instruments (2015) Endoscopy. *Product Catalog*. www.richardwolfusa.com, accessed 17 April 2015.

29. Wikipedia (2012) *Laparoscopic Surgery*. www.wikipedia.org/wiki/Laparoscopic_surgery, accessed 7 October 2012.

30. Akridge J. (2012) Operating room – high-tech surgical suites pursuing high-def tools. *Healthcare Purchasing News*, October 2012. www.hpnonline.com/inside/2012-10/1210-OR-Displays.html, accessed 17 April 2015.

31. Conmed (2015) Endosurgery. *Product Catalog*. www.conmed.com, accessed 17 April 2015.

32. Mayhew, P.D. (2013) Surgical views: thoracoscopy: basic principles, anesthetic concerns, instrumentation, and thoracic access. *Compend. Contin. Educ. Vet.*, **35**(1), E3.

33. Olympus America (2015) *Surgical Product Catalog*. www.olympusamerica.com, accessed 17 April 2015.

34. Runge, J.J. (2012) Have you attempted to de-rotate and gastropexy a GDV laparoscopically? If not … What has prevented you from doing this? 2. What is your preferred method of abdominal access, Hasson Technique or Veress Needle, and why? Vet Forum, http://vetforum.com, accessed 26 January 2013.

35. Tams, T.R. and Rawlings C.A. (2011) *Small Animal Endoscopy*, 3rd edn. Elsevier Mosby, St Louis, MO.

36. Fuller, J., Scott, W., Ashar, B., and Corrado, J. (2003) *Trocar Injuries: a Report from a U.S. Food and Drug Administration (FDA) Center for Devices and Radiological Health (CDRH) Systematic Technology Assessment of Medical Products (STAMP) Committee: FDA Safety Communication*. US Food and Drug Administration, Silver Spring, MD. http://www.fda.gov/MedicalDevices/Safety/AlertsandNotices/ucm197339.htm, accessed 17 April 2015.

37. Kolata, R. (2010) *Laparoscopic Abdominal Access and Prevention of Injury*. Ethicon Endo-Surgery, Cincinnati, OH.

38. Karl Storz (2012) *Endoscopy Product Catalogue*. www.karlstorz.com, accessed 17 April 2015.

39. Emergency Care Research Institute (ECRI) (1994) *Health Devices, Use of Wrong Gas in Laparoscopic Insufflator Causes Fire Hazard*. www.mdsr.ecri.org, accessed 8 October 2012.

40. Veit, S. (2012). The era of VATS lobectomy. In *Topics in Thoracic Surgery* (ed. Cardoso, P.), Chapter 12. InTech, Rijeka, Croatia, www.intechopen.com/books/topics-in-thoracic-surgery /the-era-of-vats-lobectomy, accessed 17 April 2015.

41. Inan, A., Sen, M., Dener, C., and Bozer, M. (2005) Comparison of direct trocar and Veress needle insertion in the performance of pneumoperitoneum in laparoscopic cholecystectomy. *Acta Chir. Belg.*, **105**(**5**), 515–518.

42. Miller, R.D., Cohen, N.H., Eriksson, L.I., Fleisher, L.A., Wiener-Kronish, J.P., and Young W.L. (eds) (2014) *Miller's Anesthesia*, 8th edn. Elsevier Saunders, Philadelphia, PA.

43. Ott, D.E. (2005) *Pneumoperitoneum: Production, Management, Effects and Consequences*. Society of Laparoendoscopic Surgeons, http://laparoscopy.blogs.com, accessed 17 April 2015.

44. Ternamian, A.M. and Deitel, M. (1999) Endoscopic threaded imaging port (EndoTIP) for laparoscopy: experience with different body weights. *Obes. Surg.*, **9**(**1**), 44–47.

45. (a)Pascoe, P.J. (2007) Thoracic surgery. In *BSAVA Manual of Canine and Feline Anaesthesia and Analgesia*, 2nd edn (ed. Seymour, S. and Duke-Novakovski, T.). British Small Animal Veterinary Association, Gloucester, Chapter 21; (b) Peláez, M. and Jolliffe, C. (2012) Thoracoscopic foreign body removal and right middle lung lobectomy to treat pyothorax in a dog. *J. Small Anim. Pract.*, **53**(**4**), 240–244.

46. Lawrentschuk, N., Fleshner, N.E., and Bolton, D.M. (2010) Laparoscopic lens fogging: a review of etiology and methods to maintain a clear visual field. *J. Endourol.*, **24**(**6**), 905–913.

SUGGESTED READING

Amann, K. and Haas, C.S. (2006) What you should know about the work-up of a renal biopsy. *Nephrol. Dial. Transplant.*, **21**(**5**), 1157–1161.

De Noto, G. (2012) *SILS™: Cholecystectomy*. Surgical Videos, www.covidien.com/covidien/videos, accessed 7 October 2012.

García, F., Prandi, D., Peña, T., Franch, J., Trasserra, O., and de la Fuente, J. (1998) Examination of the thoracic cavity and lung lobectomy by means of thoracoscopy in dogs. *Can. Vet. J.*, **39**(**5**), 285–291.

Jiménez Peláez, M., Bouvy, B.M., and Dupré, G.P. (2008) Laparoscopic adrenalectomy for treatment of unilateral adrenocortical carcinomas: technique, complications, and results in seven dogs. *Vet. Surg.*, **37**(**5**), 444–453.

Lipscomb, V.J., Hardie, R.J., and Dubielzig, R.R. (2003) Spontaneous pneumothorax caused by pulmonary blebs and bullae in 12 dogs. *J. Am. Anim. Hosp. Assoc.*, **39**(**5**), 435–445.

McCarthy, T.C. (1999) Diagnostic thoracoscopy. *Clin. Tech. Small Anim. Pract.*, **14**(**4**), 213–219.

McCarthy, T.C. (ed.) (2005) *Veterinary Endoscopy for the Small Animal Practitioner*. Elsevier Saunders, St Louis, MO.

Monnet, E. (2012) Thoracoscopy: what is possible? In *Proceedings of ACVS Veterinary Symposium 2012*. American College of Veterinary Surgeons, Germantown, MD, pp. 214–218.

Moore, A.H. and Ragni, R.A. (eds) (2012) *Clinical Manual of Small Animal Endosurgery*. Blackwell Publishing, Oxford.

Mutter, D., Garcia, A. and Jourdan, I. (2005) *Endoscopes*. WeBSurg.com, www.websurg.com/doi-ot02en308a.htm, accessed 6 October 2012.

Pizzi, R.(2009) *Diagnostic Laparoscopic Surgery in a Bush Dog*. Veterinary Laparoscopy, www.veterinarylaparoscopy.com, accessed 12 October 2012.

Plesman, R., Johnson, M., Rurak, S., Ambrose, B., and Shmon, C. (2011) Thoracoscopic correction of a congenital persistent right aortic arch in a young cat. *Can. Vet. J.*, **52**(**10**), 1123–1128.

Runge, J.J. (2011) *Thoracoscopic Pyothorax Lavage*. Vet Forum, http://vetforum.com, accessed 26 January 2013.

Runge, J.J. (2012) The cutting edge: introducing reduced port laparoscopic surgery. *Today's Vet. Pract.*, **2**(**1**), 20.

Smith, R.R., Mayhew, P.D., and Berent A.C. (2012) Laparoscopic adrenalectomy for management of a functional adrenal tumor in a cat. *J. Am. Vet. Med. Assoc.*, **241**(**3**), 368–372.

Thoracoscopy (2013). *Stedman's Medical Dictionary*. Dictionary.com, www.dictionary.reference .com/browse/thoracoscopy, accessed 2 April 2013.

Veterinary Laparoscopy (2012). *Instruments and Equipment Review*. www.vetlapsurg.com, accessed 8 October 2012.

Walsh, P.J., Remedios, A.M., Ferguson, J.F., Walker, D.D., Cantwell, S., and Duke, T. (1999) Thoracoscopic versus open partial pericardiectomy in dogs: comparison of postoperative pain and morbidity. *Vet. Surg.*, **28**(**6**), 472–479.

10 Arthroscopy

Susan Cox

William R. Pritchard Veterinary Medical Teaching Hospital, University of California-Davis, Davis, California, USA

Arthroscopy was introduced to the veterinary profession with equine medicine in the early 1970s. The first small animal procedures were performed in the late 1970s.

Arthroscopy is the use of an endoscope to examine the interior of any joint. Elbows, shoulders, and stifle joints are the most common sites. Cannulae are placed at strategic points around the joint, then the arthroscope is inserted through a cannula and into the joint, allowing for visualization. Instrument cannulae are also be positioned in the joint, allowing for more versatility.

Advantages over arthrotomy include the following:

- Magnification of the joint with the arthroscope optics
- Minimally invasive – less trauma to highly innervated joint capsule
- Shorter patient recovery time owing to smaller incisions, minimal postoperative pain, and, as a result, faster limb use.

Disadvantages include the increased knowledge base and dexterity required to perform the procedure and the cost plus repair of the equipment. Many veterinary conferences have programs for introduction to arthroscopy, but not how to assist the arthroscopist. It falls on the veterinary technician to be responsible for the equipment, to prepare the surgery, and to be the surgical assistant. Formulate anesthetic, surgical, and postsurgical plans with the arthroscopist for every patient and discuss any concerns regarding the patient or equipment.

EQUIPMENT AND INSTRUMENTATION

Arthroscopy is a surgical procedure performed in the operating room using strict aseptic techniques. It is therefore imperative that all equipment that comes in

Endoscopy for the Veterinary Technician, First Edition. Edited by Susan Cox.
© 2016 John Wiley & Sons, Inc. Published 2016 by John Wiley & Sons, Inc.

contact with the joint undergoes the sterilization process. It is important to famil-
iarize yourself with the equipment – for example, some instruments may need to
be disassembled for proper sterilization, and arthroscopes and cannulae from different manufacturers may not be compatible. Also, check with the manufacturer
for sterilization guidelines – some instruments may not be autoclavable.

The arthroscope, or rigid telescope, is the principal piece of equipment in
arthroscopy. It is also used in female cystoscopy (see Chapter 8), and rhinoscopy
(see Chapter 6). Common diameters are 2.7 and 2.4 mm, with 1.9 mm for the
carpus or tarsus. The average working length is 12 cm or shorter, although 18 cm
arthroscopes are available. Most arthroscopes used in veterinary arthroscopy
have a 30° field of view (FOV), although 0 and 70° FOVs are also available. The
working length is divided into short (8.5 cm), which is easier to handle in the
elbow, and long (13 cm), for the shoulder or knee. Because of the small diameter
and fragile fiber-optics, arthroscopes should always be used with a cannula, and
never bent within the joint. An example is shown in Figure 10.1.

The arthroscope is introduced into the joint through a cannula, which is a
hollow steel tube. The cannula supports the portal into the joint, protects the
arthroscope, and allows fluid to enter the joint space. The arthroscope and cannula lock together at the proximal end. Pictured in Figure 10.2, obturators (blunt
tip) or trocars (sharp tip) fit inside the cannula and serve as an initial "guide" into
the joint. Obturators are used most often in veterinary arthroscopy (less trauma
to cartilage).

Small-gauge hand instruments are essential to reduce trauma and increase
accuracy in the joint space. An arthroscopy pack should include a basic surgery
pack and the following instruments. Right-angle probes (Figure 10.3) have a
90° bend at the working end and are useful for scanning under bone and tissue
and retraction within the joint. Graspers have alligator-type jaws and are used
to remove bone and cartilage. Rongeurs are used much like graspers, but have

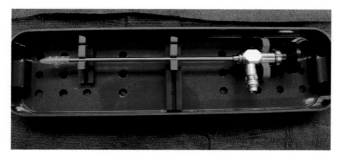

Figure 10.1 Arthroscope in autoclavable instrument tray. Light cables connect at the light
guide attachment, and a camera attaches at the eyepiece.

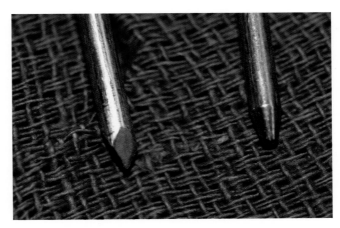

Figure 10.2 Obturator (blunt tip) and trocar (sharp tip) fit inside the cannula and establish portals into joint spaces.

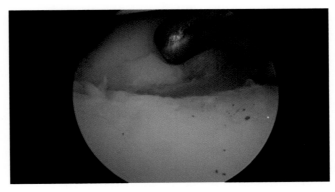

Figure 10.3 A blunt probe is viewed in elbow arthroscopy. Note the magnified image that allows for a thorough examination of the joint space.

sharp-cupped jaws to extract joint tissue. Opened and closed types of curettes should also be included for debriding cartilage or bone (see Figure 10.4). There are many other types of hand instruments that may be added to the arthroscopy pack – for more information, see Suggested reading.

A power shaver is a motorized tool that removes bone cartilage and soft tissue swiftly and accurately. A disposable shaver bit is attached to the handpiece. The handpiece is attached to a control box, which acts as the power supply. The forward or backward oscillations of the bit are controlled from the handle or with a foot pedal. The bits are housed inside a beveled cannula and may be changed

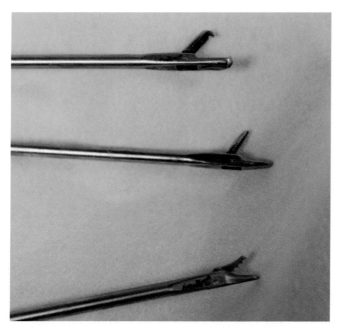

Figure 10.4 The working end of three types of forceps: from top to bottom, punch forceps with hook, retrieval forceps, and scissors forceps.

according to the procedure being performed. The bit cannula also has a suction attachment to remove small pieces of joint tissue that the shaver debrides. Make sure that the bit housing is dry before assembly.

An arthroscope being used in elbow arthroscopy is shown in Figure 10.6. Because of the large amount of fluid exchange, a plastic drape is recommended and should cover the entire patient. The surgical endoscopist creates a fenestration over the surgical site, as pictured in Figure 10.7. The plastic material helps to avoid contamination from saturated paper or cloth drapes.

Radiofrequency and electrocautery units are also used to cauterize blood vessels and as tissue-ablating tools within the joint space. They are available as bipolar and monopolar types. The unit includes a control box, foot pedal, and handpiece with tip.

A fluid pathway must be established for visualization within the joint. Blood and tissue debris can cloud the small viewing area, so 0.9% saline or lactated Ringer's solution must be constantly exchanged. Fluid infusion also distends the joint, allowing for a broader viewing zone, so an ingress and egress fluid system is necessary. Cannulae possess a port to attach the fluid administration set for fluid ingress. If an arthroscopy procedure is known to be prolonged at the outset, large 3–5 L fluid bags inside fluid compression bags (as shown in Figure 10.5) may be

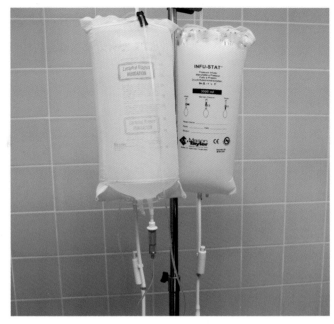

Figure 10.5 Large-volume fluid bags inside compression bags for joint flush. A sterile extension set is attached to the infusion set and also to the ingress system.

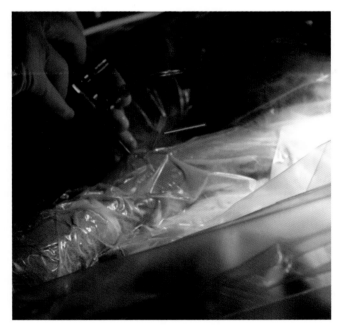

Figure 10.6 An arthroscope being used in elbow arthroscopy, with an 18 Fr needle (blue arrow) used as fluid egress. The patient is in left lateral recumbency.

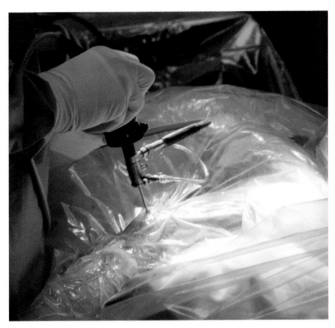

Figure 10.7 The arthroscope in the joint space, with the cranial end of the patient towards the lower right of the image. The clear fluid line and light cable are attached to the sheath.

considered. Fluid pumps are also available and can deliver fluid at a steady set rate, which can be useful when power shavers are utilized.

A camera head that can be sterilized is necessary for arthroscopy. The camera is attached to the arthroscope via a C-clamp at the eyepiece. A sterile light cable is also attached to the arthroscope at the light guide port. Ports and attachments on the light cable and arthroscope vary among manufacturers, so light cable adapters may be needed for a secure attachment. Most camera heads on the market feature buttons that control white balance, along with video and image capture. Check with the manufacturer for sterilization guidelines.

The camera box, light source, image capture, shaver control box, and optional fluid pump and electrocautery unit should be kept on a mobile component tower. The tower should have a swing arm mount for a medical-grade video monitor, and be equipped with movable shelves and large wheels for positioning in the operating room.

Aids for positioning the joint are available commercially, or can be custommade according to the arthroscopist's preference, as shown in Figure 10.8. Vacuum bean-bag positioners can aid in maintaining a dog in the desired position.

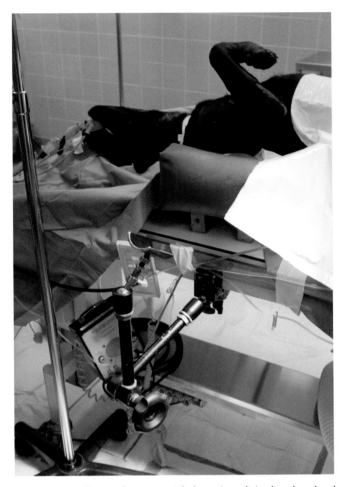

Figure 10.8 Positioners for elbow arthroscopy. A bolster (in red) is placed under the elbow joint. A custom-made elbow positioner holds the thoracic limb in pronation, which opens the joint space.

An equipment list is given in Box 10.1.

BOX 10.1 EQUIPMENT LIST.

- Component tower
  - Video monitor on swing arm
  - Camera box
  - Light source
  - Image capture device
  - Power shaver box
  - Fluid pump

- ○ Electrofrequency and electrocautery units
- Sterile camera
- Sterile light cable
- Suction pump with sterile suction tubing
- Plastic barrier drape
- Positioning aids
  - ○ Vacuum bean-bag positioner
  - ○ Limb positioners
- Absorbent pads secured to floor
- Arthroscope
  - ○ 2.7 or 2.4 mm most common
- Cannula
  - ○ Trocar – sharp tip
  - ○ Obturator – blunt tip
- Fluids
  - ○ Lactated Ringer's solution – two 3 or 5 L bags
  - ○ Saline 0.9% – two 3 or 5 L bags
- Shavers
  - ○ Disposable cutting bits – 2.5–4.0 mm in diameter
  - ○ Burr bits – 2.5–4.0 mm in diameter
- Basic surgical pack
  - ○ Surgical blade – arthroscopist preference
  - ○ Bowl with saline and 12 mL syringes
  - ○ Six 1 1/2 in 18 or 22 French gauge (Fr) needles
  - ○ Non-absorbable suture – arthroscopist preference
- Basic hand instruments set
  - ○ 90° hooked probe
  - ○ Graspers
  - ○ Arthroscopic rongeurs
  - ○ Curettes – 2–3 mm in diameter
    - ■ Opened
    - ■ Closed
  - ○ Arthroscopic scissors – 2–3 mm in diameter
  - ○ Osteotome – 2–3 mm in diameter

PATIENT PREPARATION

In addition to the minimum database, patients undergoing arthroscopy may require preoperative computed tomography (CT), radiographs, and/or joint ultrasound to evaluate the affected joint properly prior to arthroscopy. These procedures may need to be performed after anesthetic induction, and should be factored into the anesthetic plan.

A wide clip of the affected limb is recommended. Rotation or manipulation of the joint may be necessary, or an arthrotomy may instead be the best course of action. Wrapping and suspending the distal portion of the affected limb can aid

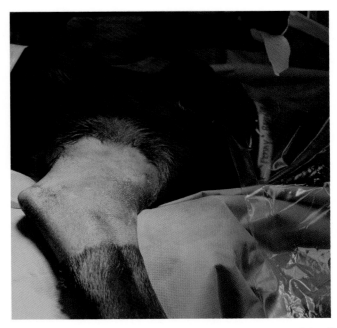

Figure 10.9 Elbow joints are prepared for arthroscopy. The medial aspect of the elbow is clipped and prepped with alternating chlorhexidine scrub and 70% alcohol on 4 × 4 gauze sponges. The area is prepped in the OR with sterile gloves, gauze, and zepharin and allowed to remain for 3 min before draping.

in the surgical preparation. A preliminary surgical scrub should be performed, with a final prep in the operating room (OR).

As in Figure 10.9, both joints (i.e. elbows) may need arthroscopy. All additional draping and surgical materials should be on hand to reduce operative and anesthesia turnaround time for the patient.

PREPARATION OF THE SURGICAL SUITE

The OR should be arranged so that the arthroscopist can easily see the video monitor during surgery. The overhead lights are off in order to visualize the monitor better. The tower should also be accessible for camera and light-guide connections. The surgical endoscopist or the assistant should have foot controls within reach. Absorbent padding can be taped to the floor to soak up saline and prevent slipping. The surgical table should be able to tilt, and move lower or higher at the arthroscopist's request. Positioning aids must also be securely attached to the table. A typical room arrangement is shown in Figures 10.10 and 10.11.

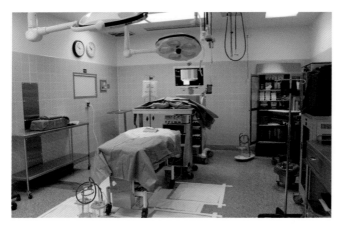

Figure 10.10 The OR is prepared for arthroscopy. Absorbent pads are taped on the floor to catch fluids. The monitor tower is positioned behind the instrument table. An additional instrument table holds video equipment, shaver handles, and instruments.

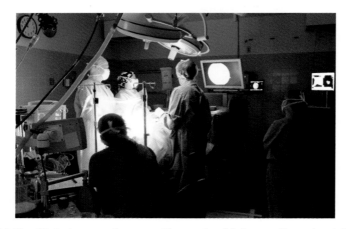

Figure 10.11 The OR during an arthroscopy. The overhead lights are dimmed and the monitor is placed for easy viewing from all angles. The CT images are also available (right side of image) for reference.

GENERAL ARTHROSCOPY

- General anesthesia
- Clip and preliminary surgical prep affected limb
  - Wrap paw and suspend from pole if needed
  - Prep technician masked and examination gloves worn
- Transfer to OR
- Remove leg from pole and place in position
- Final surgical prep

- Patient draped/surgical instruments arranged
- Stab incisions at cannula placement sites
- Distend joint before cannula placement
  - 1 1/2 in 22 Fr needle placed at portal site
  - 6–15 mL of 0.9% saline instilled
  - Plunger will back out of the syringe when the joint is adequately distended
  - Remove needle
- Place cannula with trocar
  - Remove trocar and advance cannula when joint space entered
- Insert arthroscope and lock onto cannula
- Attach fluid line
  - Allow fluid to redistend joint before examining
  - Place egress needle if needed for fluid exchange
- Orient camera and arthroscope within joint
  - Establishes left and right direction
  - Anatomic references
    - Elbow – anconeal process
    - Shoulder – biceps tendon
    - Stifle – intercondylar notch
- Explore joint
  - Identify problems
  - Perform appropriate procedure
  - Additional instrument portal may be needed
- Redistend and irrigate joint
  - Flush and remove any tissue/bone debris
- Remove instrumentation
- Suture incision(s)
- Encourage endoscopist to complete surgery report.

ELBOW ARTHROSCOPY

- Dorsal recumbency for medial approach
- Prepare affected elbow(s)
  - Clip mid-metacarpus to mid-humerus
  - Wrap paw/exposed fur
  - Preliminary scrub
  - Transfer to OR
- Position according to arthroscopist's requirements
  - Sandbags lateral to elbows
  - Custom positioners – see Figure 10.8
    - Pronate elbow to open joint (valgus stress)
    - Tape lower leg to positioner to hold in pronation (see Figure 10.12)

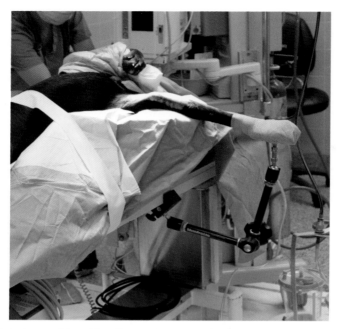

Figure 10.12 Patient positioned for elbow arthroscopy. The dog is placed in the ventro-dorsal position with the left elbow secured to the positioner for a medial approach. A plastic drape is placed over the entire patient.

- Final prep in OR
- Joint distension with saline
- Portal placement(s)
- Indications and treatment
  - Fragmented medial coronoid process (FCP)
    - Identified as
      - Defective cartilage fragment, as shown in Figure 10.13
    - Treatment
      - Subtotal coronoidectomy
        - CT can aid in visualization of fragment
        - Removal of abnormal tissue fragment
          - Use shaver, or osteotome to break up large fragment, graspers to remove pieces
        - Power shave/curette coronoid to smooth surface
        - Microfracture to encourage fibrocartilage and healing
        - Examine joint for missed pieces
        - Flush all debris out of joint
        - Remove instrumentation, suture incision(s)

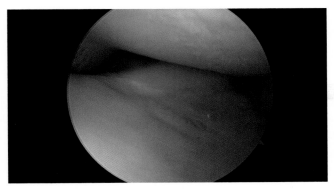

Figure 10.13 Fragmented medial coronoid process revealed during elbow arthroscopy. The fragment was elevated with a blunt probe as in Figure 10.3 and removed with grasping forceps.

- Instruments required for removal of fragment
  - Power shaver unit
  - Curette
  - Alligator graspers
  - Osteotome
  - 70° microfracture pick
- Postsurgical patient care – check with arthroscopist for guidelines
  - Pain control
  - No bandage needed
  - Cold therapy
    - Reduce pain and swelling
    - Ice packs on elbow
  - Exercise restriction
  - Recheck appointments
- Osteochondritis dissecans (OCD)
  - Affects large dog breeds
  - Identified as
    - Loose cartilage flap at the medial portion of the left lateral condyle
  - Treatment
    - Flap removal with graspers
    - Debridement with curette or power shaver
    - Microfracture to encourage fibrocartilage and healing
    - Saline flush
    - Remove instrumentation, suture incisions
  - Instrumentation – same as for FCP
  - Postsurgical patient care – same as for FCP

- ○ Ununited anconeal process
  - Primarily young canines
  - Failure of unification of anconeus with the proximal ulna
  - Concurrent FCP in many patients
  - Treatment
    - − Correct FCP
    - − Assess joint; arthroscope can assist with arthrotomy correction if warranted
- ○ Neoplasia
  - Synovial sarcomas most common
  - Abnormal tissue visualized and biopsied with cup biopsy forceps.

SHOULDER ARTHROSCOPY

- General anesthesia
- Lateral recumbency
- Clip beyond scapula and below elbow, as shown in Figure 10.15
- Wrap leg to elbow, then surgical scrub
- Transport to OR
- Unilateral arthroscopy
  - ○ Surgeon and assistant on one side of the table with tower opposite
- Bilateral arthroscopy
  - ○ Tower beyond instrument table
  - ○ Other shoulder clipped; surgical prep performed when turned
- Affected shoulder in neutral position, as in Figures 10.14 and 10.15
  - ○ Parallel to floor
  - ○ Support with Mayo stand, limb positioner(s)
- Drape patient and prepare instruments
- Egress portal established
  - ○ Egress cannula or $1\,{}^1\!/_2$ in 16–18 Fr needle placed first
  - ○ Joint fluid sample obtained if warranted
- Joint distended with 0.9% saline or LRS through egress
- Assistant holds syringe plunger while arthroscope portal and fluid ingress are established
- Instrument portal placed
- Orient camera to monitor in joint
- Assistant may need to rotate limb to allow full shoulder joint visualization
- Explore joint
  - ○ Identify problems
  - ○ Perform appropriate procedure
- Redistend and irrigate joint
  - ○ Flush and remove any tissue/bone debris

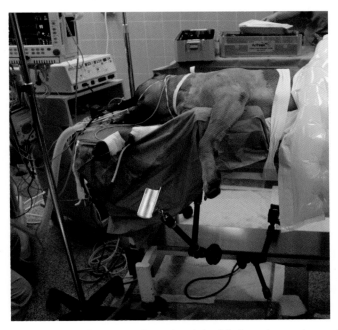

Figure 10.14 Left shoulder arthroscopy. The patient is in right lateral recumbency. Positioning aids are the same as for elbow arthroscopy.

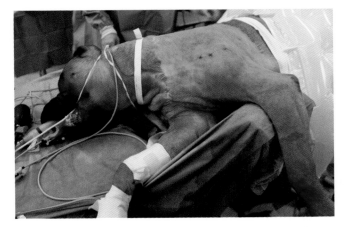

Figure 10.15 Postsurgical shoulder arthroscopy patient. Note the incisions demonstrating port placements. A wide clip beyond the scapula is also shown.

- Remove instrumentation
- Suture incision(s)
- Indications
  ○ Osteochondritis dissecans

- Cartilage fragment lifted from articular surface
  - Can be completely detached and free-floating
- Often bilateral
  ○ Instrumentation
    - 2.7 or 2.4 mm arthroscope
    - Alligator grasper
    - Probe
    - Instrument cannula
    - Power shaver/curette
    - Options
      - Radiofrequency device
      - Fluid pump
  ○ Treatment
    - Lift flap with probe
    - Leave small attachment at site; remove probe
    - Alligator forceps to remove flap
      - May need to remove in pieces in older dog
    - Debride all loose cartilage
      - Power shaver or curette
    - Irrigate joint
      - Flush and remove any tissue/bone debris
    - Remove instrumentation
    - Suture incision(s)
  ○ Postsurgical patient care
    - Restrict activity for 4–6 weeks or clinician recommendation
- Biceps tenosynovitis
  ○ Indications
    - Partial tear of the biceps tendon
  ○ Instrumentation
    - 2.7 or 2.4 mm arthroscope
    - Probe
    - Instrument cannula
    - No. 15 surgical blade with handle
    - Radiofrequency unit
    - Fluid pump
  ○ Treatment
    - Instrument portal placed medial or lateral to the biceps tendon
    - 1 1/2 in 22 Fr needle at proximal aspect of biceps tendon, either medial or lateral

- Scalpel blade inserted into joint and cuts tendon near needle, or radiofrequency unit through instrument portal to transect tendon
  - Irrigate joint
    - Flush and remove any debris
  - Remove instrumentation
  - Suture incision(s), as shown in Figure 10.15
  - ○ Postsurgical patient care
    - Restrict exercise for 4 weeks
  - ○ Neoplasia
  - ○ Joint examined
  - ○ Samples procured with arthroscopic biopsy forceps
    - Irrigate joint
      - Flush and remove any debris
    - Remove instrumentation
  - ○ Suture incision(s).

STIFLE ARTHROSCOPY

- Indications
  - ○ Cranial cruciate ligament stump debridement prior to stabilization
  - ○ Examination of meniscus
    - Removal of torn sections
  - ○ OCD debridement
  - ○ Biopsy
    - Intra-articular neoplasia
    - Synovial membrane
  - ○ Evaluation of the stifle joint
- General anesthesia
  - ○ Discontinue aspirin therapy 1 week before procedure
  - ○ Epidural performed (clinician preference)
- Clip from mid-metatarsus to hip joint
- Wrap paw, suspend limb (arthroscopist preference), surgical scrub, transfer to OR
- Dorsal recumbency
  - ○ Cranial end of table tilted (arthroscopist preference)
  - ○ Arthroscopist and assistant working at end of table
  - ○ Instrument table over patient
  - ○ Tower at tableside
  - ○ Vacuum bean-bag device helpful to hold patient
- Drape patient and prepare instruments

- Instruments
  - 2.7 mm arthroscope
  - Power shaver unit
  - Electrofrequency unit
  - Fluid pump
  - Probe, graspers, biopsy forceps, curettes
- Establish portals, fluid ingress/egress cannulae or needles
- Stifle joint examined
  - Assistant may need to flex/extend limb for optimal visualization of all areas
    - Valgus stress
    - Flexion
    - External rotation
- Elected treatment performed
- Joint flushed and final inspection
  - Intra-articular bupivacaine injected if epidural not performed (clinician preference)
    - Egress cannula/needle can be used
- Incisions closed
- Arthrotomy performed, or patient awakened
- Postoperative care
  - Robert Jones bandage placed on affected limb for 12–24 h
  - Cold therapy
  - NSAIDs, opioids, fentanyl patch (clinician preference)
  - Weight control (long-term)
  - Exercise restriction; cage rest
- Encourage surgical endoscopist to complete surgical report.

SAMPLE COLLECTION AND PROCESSING

Joint fluid, if collected in a sterile manner, can be submitted for cytologic evaluation or placed on a culturette swab for anaerobic culture. Samples of joint tissue may be collected and placed in labeled formalin jars for evaluation.

COMPLICATIONS

Swelling may be seen at the surgical site from subcutaneous fluid buildup from fluid exchange. A Robert Jones bandage placed on elbows or stifles for 24 h may be beneficial. An example is shown in Figure 10.16. Extracapsular fluid buildup after shoulder arthroscopy should resorb in 24 h. Implant failure or migration (ununited anconeal process, fractures) may occur and need to be addressed.

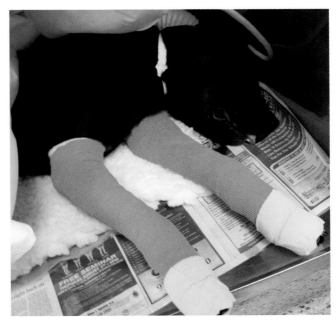

Figure 10.16 Support bandages are placed after elbow arthroscopy and while the patient is under anesthesia. Bandages are (hopefully) left on overnight.

ACKNOWLEDGMENT

The author would like to thank the Small Animal Orthopedic Service at the UC Davis VMTH for their assistance with this chapter.

SUGGESTED READING

Beale, B.S., Hulse, D.A., Schulz, K., and Whitney, W.O. (2003) *Small Animal Arthroscopy*. W.B. Saunders, Philadelphia, PA.

Tams, T.R. and Rawlings, C.A. (eds) (2011) *Small Animal Endoscopy*, 3rd edn. Elsevier Mosby, St Louis, MO, pp. 607–621.

11 The ultimate endoscopy suite

Susan Cox

William R. Pritchard Veterinary Medical Teaching Hospital, University of California-Davis, Davis,California, USA

Healthcare facilities are continuously constructing state-of-the-art endoscopy rooms to keep up with high patient demand and changes in endoscopic technology. Although a dedicated endoscopy and reprocessing unit would be prohibitively expensive for most veterinary hospitals, taking a few objectives and adapting them for the veterinary profession will increase efficiency and decrease repair costs.

The ultimate endoscopy suite is comprised of two rooms:

1 Endoscopy procedure room – the procedure room has to be adaptable for all endoscopy procedures. Mobile carts that house procedural supplies and endoscopy components for transport to the point-of-care are all housed here.
2 Reprocessing room – after the endoscope has been initially cleaned (channels tested and flushed) at table-side, the endoscope and other related instruments are transported here for thorough cleaning and disinfection.

THE ENDOSCOPY PROCEDURE ROOM

Ideally, the endoscopy room should be located in the interior of the building with no windows. Close access to emergency services or ICU should also be considered, since procedures such as bronchoscopy can be performed on critical patients. A small emergency cart (see Figure 11.1) placed within easy reach is mandatory. The cart should be stocked and inspected on a regular basis. Hospital-grade electrical plugs should also be spaced around the room – near the floor and at desk height.

Surfaces, including floors, walls, counters, and workstations, should be easy to clean and disinfect. Components should be simple to move and/or disassemble

Endoscopy for the Veterinary Technician, First Edition. Edited by Susan Cox.
© 2016 John Wiley & Sons, Inc. Published 2016 by John Wiley & Sons, Inc.

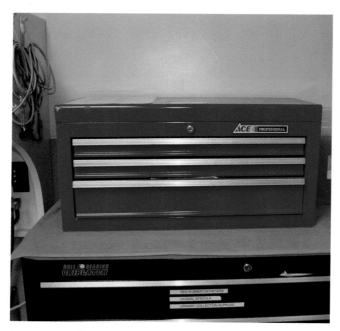

Figure 11.1 The emergency box in the endoscopy room of the William R. Pritchard Veterinary Medical Teaching Hospital at UC Davis. It is situated between two procedure tables, so is easily accessible in critical situations. Emergency drugs are kept in the top drawer that lifts up for easy access. endotracheal tubes, laryngoscope, Ambu bag, and other essentials are also kept here.

in order to clean parts easily. Elements that can gather dirt and dust, such as decorative moldings or other non-essential horizontal work surfaces should be discouraged. Wall coverings that cannot be wiped down should also be avoided. Sharps containers and biohazard receptacles should be positioned around the room for easy access.

A medical-grade video monitor shown in Figure 11.2 can be mounted on the wall or from the ceiling on an articulated arm specifically designed to support medical equipment. This invites group participation in the endoscopy procedure and is an effective use of vertical space. It also alleviates the problem of tripping or rolling over video cords. The monitor can also be rotated, depending on the endoscopy performed. Components such as video processors, light sources, and video capture equipment can also be housed on a similar swing-arm tower that includes adjustable shelving.

A wheeled tower with adjustable shelving can be an alternative. This allows endoscopy to become mobile and adds flexibility. The endoscopy tower can be available for patients that are critical and cannot be moved, or if the tower is needed in the operating room for a sterile procedure. Most mobile endoscopy towers made today have a swing arm that accommodates the monitor and

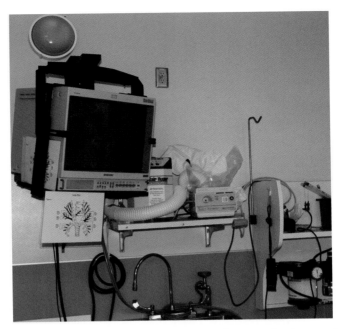

Figure 11.2 A medical-grade video monitor hung on a wall-mounted swing arm. This monitor can be swiveled so it can be viewed from any angle of the table. A bronchial diagram is affixed to the front of the monitor for reference during bronchoscopy. Shelves for heating pads (center) and anesthesia equipment make use of vertical space.

adjustable shelves for varying heights of components (Figure 11.3). The back of endoscopy carts have a door that allows access to video port connections. This feature becomes important as connections can detach when the carts are pushed through doorways and over rough surfaces. Cart options include housing for a nitrogen tank used in laparoscopies, a slide-out keyboard shelf and attachment for an IV pole. A hospital-grade outlet strip should be used with the components, as well as heavy-duty cord wraps.

Mobile procedure carts are another important feature in the endoscopy room. These carts hold items specific to a certain procedure, such as cystoscopy or gastroscopy (see Figure 11.4). Cystoscopy, for example, uses small sterile items such as biopsy cover ports and guidewire introducers that should be kept in one cart, as pictured in Figure 11.5. Carts can be transported out of the room or easily relocated to point-of-care in other areas of the hospital, or to tableside in the procedure room for endoscopy. General supply carts can also be used to house items that are used for every procedure – examination gloves, biopsy equipment, syringes, gauze, lap pads, etc. These carts should have a flat top for biopsy sampling and recording findings.

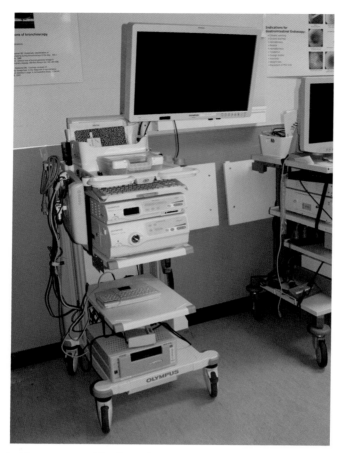

Figure 11.3 A video tower capable of traveling to other parts of the hospital. Set-up includes components for video and all-fiber-optic endoscope and telescope capability, and also adapters for different manufacturers' endoscopes. An image capture device is also included. The monitor is on a swing arm attached to the cart.

Depending on the procedure and clinician preference, endoscopy patients have to be oriented relative to the video monitor. A mobile procedure table/gurney with sturdy lockable wheels can be used to rotate the patient. Gurneys should also be height adjustable and sturdy to accommodate large dogs. Because of the turning radius of the table, the floor around the area should be kept clear. The anesthesia machine is moved with the table. An alternative to the gurney would be a grated table station attached to a sink, which would allow easy postprocedure cleanup.

Lighting in the endoscopy room can be challenging. Endoscopy monitors are best observed in a dark room. Conversely, working with small biopsy samples and anesthesia monitoring requires a degree of light to perform the

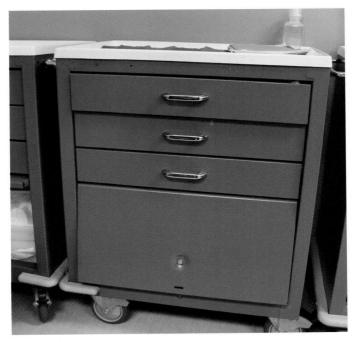

Figure 11.4 An example of a mobile storage cart for procedures. These carts have sturdy wheels and are used for multiprocedural items such as examination gloves, suction canisters, syringes, and biopsy sampling accessories.

tasks. Task lighting over workstations, including swing-arm overhead surgical and under-cabinet lights, can be directed away from the field-of-view of the endoscopist.

Several workstations should be placed around the procedure room. A small desk with a telephone, computer, and laboratory forms is practical for reviewing patient history, digital radiographs, and completing endoscopy reports. A microscope station (see Figure 11.6) is also necessary for generating, staining, and reviewing impression smears or cytology slides during and after a procedure. A two-headed teaching microscope encourages group participation.

Storage is an ongoing issue for any veterinary clinic, so it would be practical to utilize wall space and install adjustable cabinets and shelves for suction canisters, forceps, endoscope accessories, etc. Supply carts can be easily restocked from the cabinets to avoid shortages. Label the outside of each cabinet so that items can be found and removed quickly.

All endoscopes (except ultra-thins) should be stored vertically and safely. A protective cabinet should be tall enough to hang the longest endoscopes, without the endoscopes' insertion tubes touching the cabinet floor. They should be securely supported as shown in Figure 11.7 and enclosed/locked to prevent

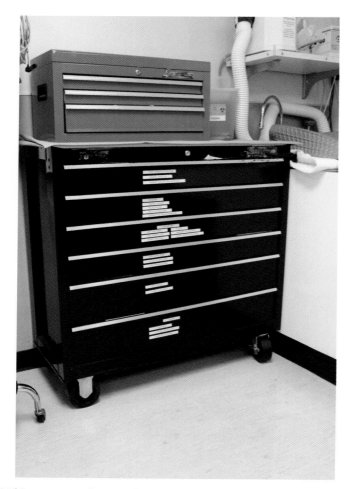

Figure 11.5 This storage cart features elongated drawers for several types of urinary catheters, and deep drawers for 0.9% saline bottles and liter fluid bags, plus other cystoscopy equipment.

accidental damage or tampering. Doors must not pose a risk for pinching endoscope insertion tubes.

Suction units can vary depending on number of endoscope procedures done and usage in other parts of the hospital. Installing centralized suction equipment with wall outlets (see Figure 11.8) in necessary rooms may be the most practical. Mobile suction units on wheels are a viable alternative.

A light box for viewing radiographs or a large screen for examining digital images should be included in the room. The light box can also provide a source of ambient light if needed.

A large, deep sink is also necessary. It serves many purposes – hand-washing, storing ice for procedures, prerinsing soiled equipment, etc.

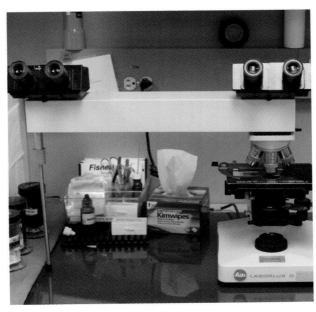

Figure 11.6 A microscope station is needed for cytologic evaluation, especially in a teaching setting. Glass slides and staining equipment are next to the microscope and close to the sink. The microscope pictured here takes about 2 ft of counter space.

Optional Equipment

Cages for pre- and postprocedure patients may provide a more secure area for observation, especially with multiple procedures scheduled. Cages with lockable wheels can be rolled in or out of the room when necessary. Be aware that rhinoscopy patients will have epistaxis with possible sneezing episodes and should have a clear area around the front of the cage.

Interventional radiology techniques utilizing fluoroscopy are occasionally guided by endoscopic modalities, especially in cystoscopy and tracheoscopy stent placement procedures. Depending on state or government standards, the procedure room must be retrofitted with the appropriate shielding materials and personnel provided with the required protective equipment. Radiation badges must also be provided.

A laundry container should be in place for soiled linens and towels and emptied on a regular basis. Several may be necessary to keep items used on infectious patients separate.

ENDOSCOPE AND INSTRUMENT PROCESSING ROOM

Depending on daily endoscope usage, endoscope cleaning and high-level disinfection can affect the timing and efficiency of a busy schedule of procedures.

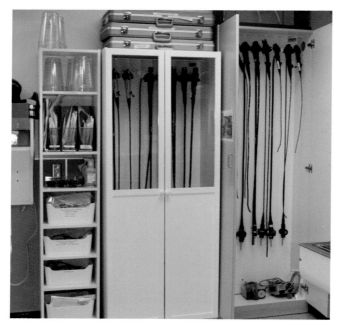

Figure 11.7 Endoscopy storage cabinets at the VMTH. An endoscope rack is attached to the inside of a long cabinet. The endoscopes are placed high enough so that the insertion tubes do not touch the cabinet floor. Water bottles, suction canisters, and flexible biopsy and retrieval forceps are stored adjacent to the endoscopes so that related items can be kept in one location.

Ideally, endoscope processing rooms should be adjacent to the procedure room. This allows better flow of endoscopes and instrumentation from the contaminated area to the clean area and ultimately to storage or back in use for the next procedure. As in the procedure room, surfaces should be easy to clean and sanitize.

Endoscope cleaning requires large volumes of water and is a wet area. Oversized sinks are handy for leak testing and cleaning gross material from the endoscope and accessories. Adequate counter space should be available to accommodate a "dirty" area (usually next to the sink) and a "clean" area, as shown in Figure 11.9. The "dirty" area holds postprocedure endoscopes (tableside precleaning/flushing has already been performed) and other used instrumentation. Endoscopes are brushed and flushed in this area prior to high-level disinfection. The clean area will hold endoscopes directly out of the endoscope reprocessor or soaking tray. A small ultrasonic cleaner should be included in the room to clean forceps and small items. A line of GFCI (ground-fault circuit interrupter) electrical outlets should also be installed.

Depending on caseload and endoscope usage, installing an automated endoscope reprocessor may be a valuable asset in the clinic. They decrease

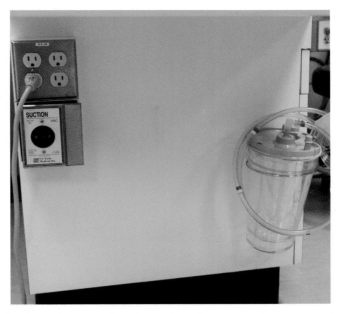

Figure 11.8 Suction outlet port and suction canister. The port attachment connects from the outlet port to the canister lid port. Separate tubing connects to the endoscope's suction port on the terminal end. These ports can be placed in the clinic wherever suction may be needed.

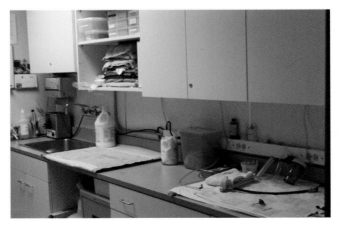

Figure 11.9 A long counter in the endoscope processing room is divided into the "dirty" side and the "clean" side. In the upper left side of the image plastic containers hold separate cleaning brushes for each endoscope. Ample storage cabinets hold additional endoscopy equipment such as PEG tubes and balloon dilators. An ultrasonic cleaner is placed near the sink.

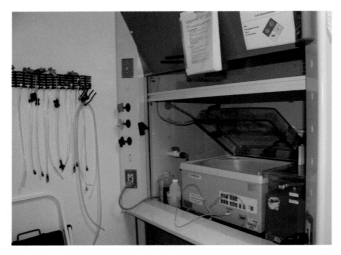

Figure 11.10 An automated endoscope reprocessor in a fume hood. The tank adjacent to the reprocessor houses the high-level disinfection solution. UV and water filters are also connected within the water lines attached to the tub of the reprocessor. Rubber mat pieces attached to the wall neatly hold tubing that connects the endoscope to the reprocessor.

exposure to disinfection solutions and save time by automatically washing, disinfecting, and rinsing all channels of the endoscope and instrumentation. Several endoscope companies also manufacture automated reprocessors, as shown in Figure 11.10.

Storage cabinets, drawers, and shelving can be useful to house accessories such as extra biopsy forceps, disinfection solution, and personal protective equipment (PPE) for fluoroscopy and laser lithotripsy. Wider cabinets can hold ultrathin or flexible cystoscopes in their cases.

A forced-air system can be invaluable to dry an endoscope's channels in a short period of time. Medical air compressors can be installed for whole-hospital use with outlet ports. Flexible silicone tubing can be adapted to fit onto endoscope ports as endoscopes are drying after high-level disinfection, either on the counter or hanging against the wall, as shown in Figure 11.11. This ensures that all moisture is removed from the endoscope. A commercial-grade air filter should be installed inline and replaced according to the manufacturer's specifications.

Optional equipment to complete the endoscopy suite could be an icemaker, used for vasoconstriction in rhinoscopies and cystoscopies. A warming cabinet for warming IV fluids and saline bottles used in bronchoscopies can also be helpful.

Organizing a complete work space dedicated to endoscopy, such as in Figure 11.12, can be a major undertaking. Having the correct tools within reach keeps the endoscopist happy and makes the procedure go smoothly for you and the patient.

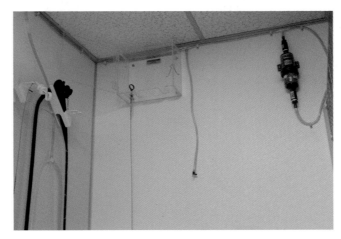

Figure 11.11 A forced-air system winds around the reprocessing room. Tubing is directed to the "clean side" of the counter for preliminary forced-air action, and at several endoscope hanger stations for an additional 15–20 min. Many endoscope hangers include areas to hang biopsy forceps for thorough drying.

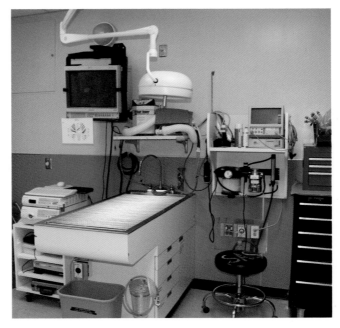

Figure 11.12 One of the endoscopy procedure tables at the VMTH. Ambient light is provided using dimmers on wall lights (above the monitor). Focused task lighting is accomplished with surgical lights on swing arms. A table with a removal grate top is easy to clean. The component tower is mobile to accommodate any endoscopy procedure.

SUGGESTED READING

Department of Veterans Affairs, Office of Construction and Facilities Management (2011) *Design Guide: Digestive Diseases – Endoscopy Service*. www.cfm.va.gov/til/dGuide/dgDigestiveEndoscopy .pdf, accessed 18 April 2015.

EndoNurse (2005) *Endoscopy Suite*. www.endonurse.com/articles/2005/02/endoscopy-suite .aspx, accessed 18 April 2015.

Herman Miller Inc., Endoscopy Department (1999) *Graphic Standards Programming and Schematic Design*. www.facilityresources.ca/healthcare/endoscopy.pdf, accessed 18 April 2015.

Index

Page numbers in *italics* refer to figures; those in **bold** to tables.

Endoscopy for the Veterinary Technician, First Edition. Edited by Susan Cox.
© 2016 John Wiley & Sons, Inc. Published 2016 by John Wiley & Sons, Inc.